THE OBESITY:

Multiple Choice Questions

Learn & Prepare

FOURTH EDITION

Muhammad Asad MD

Author

Muhammad Asad MD, FACS, FASMBS

Bariatric and Minimally Invasive Surgeon

Diplomate American Board of Obesity Medicine

Contents

Foreword

With great excitement, this edition of "The Obesity: Multiple Choice Questions" is coming to a reality. The content of the book is structured to enhance understanding of the subject and give the reader an edge on preparation for certification. Top authorities have written the questions in the field of Obesity Medicine. These experts not only are actively engaged in their fields but also are clinicians and teachers with decades of experience. The questions are objectively crafted and focus on key areas of current interest. The content of the problem based multiple-choice questions focuses on the most relevant issues in the subject of obesity and emphasizes a multidimensional approach to deal with this national epidemic.

The authors of this book have spent a vast amount of time developing these questions from their clinical practices. They have done extensive research on what are the most current and relevant topics about Obesity. This book can provide the tools necessary to enhance understanding the mechanisms and management principles underlying the disease process. The fourth edition is a collaboration of many clinicians who contributed their enthusiasm and motivation. Their helpful and valuable insight gives this fourth edition a respectable place in the available publications for review of bariatric medicine.

I feel this book will help healthcare providers better know about obesity. It will give them wisdom and knowledge to become better practicing clinicians.

Asif Shakoor MD
UPMC Hamot Erie, PA, USA

Preface

This is the fourth edition of Obesity Multiple Choice Questions book. Management of obesity is a rapidly expanding discipline. A growing number of physicians and allied staff are interested in learning about this serious and alarming health problem. There is a sizeable literature available, and it is expanding. Recommendations and standards of care are constantly evolving. It is important to continue to move forward with a regular update cycle of this manuscript to keep it relevant. Main objective is not only to provide a resource for preparation for the examination, but more so to make it a problem-based learning tool for the healthcare professionals. In this latest iteration many questions are revised. Cues from actual clinical cases are transformed into problem-based scenarios. New explanations are added.

A self-assessment exam is now available based on the content of this book. A separate publication now exists by the author on subject of obesity related pharmacology.

I feel this book will be a valuable contribution to the existing literature. Questions derived from actual clinical problems will help the readers fill gaps in understanding and improve knowledge to become better clinicians.

Passion to learn and teach is the driving force for me and my colleagues to keep moving this work forward. It may not be a perfect book, but I am certain that we are in the right direction. Limited time and resources for this kind of endeavor are not holding us back. I appreciate help of all team members.

Muhammad Asad FACS, FASMBS
Diplomate American Board of Obesity Medicine

Contributors

Irtaza Asar
Attending Physician EM, Saint Vincent Hospital Erie, PA, USA
Hana Manzoor MD
Resident Internal Medicine, Beaumont Hospital Dearborn, MI
Avais Raja MD
Resident Internal Medicine, Beaumont Hospital Dearborn, MI
Marhaba Mabroor Fatima Medical Student, University of Buckingham, Buckingham, UK
Muhammad Anshaal Muneeb Chawdhery
Medical Student, Medical University, Sofia, Bulgaria

Disclaimer

Although every possible precaution has been made to ensure the accuracy of the information contained in this book, the authors and publisher assume no responsibility for any errors or omissions. No liability is assumed for damages that may result from the use of information contained in this publication.

The Scope of The Problem

Question 1.1

Obesity is recognized as one of the major health issues in recent years. Select the correct statement.

a. Emphasis on avoiding fat has led to an increased consumption of carbohydrates

b. Larger food volumes over the course of last few decades

c. More sedentary lifestyle changes

d. High carbohydrate diets and the presence of insulin resistance contribute to significant weight gain

e. All the above statements are correct

The correct answer is "e."

In recent years, obesity has become as one of the significant health issues in developed and developing nations. The components leading to the development of obesity are recognized to be high carbohydrate diets, larger portion sizes, and sedentary lifestyles. In patients with insulin resistance, high carbohydrate-containing foods can lead to significant weight gain. Drinking one regular soda daily may lead to a gain of 10 to 15 pounds of weight in one year.
"Overweight & Obesity." Centers for Disease Control and Prevention, Centers for Disease Control and Prevention, 13 Aug. 2018, www.cdc.gov/obesity/data/adult.html.

Question 1.2

What is the prevalence of obesity in US according to Statistics from the Center for Disease Control and Prevention (CDC) (2017 to 18)?

a. 16.4%

b. 19.4%

c. 26.4%

d. 31.4%

e. 42.4%

The correct answer is "e."

Prevalence of obesity in US has gone up in recent years. Changing lifestyles and eating behaviors are the main contributing factors. Estimations show that now 42.4 % of US population is obese. Non-Hispanic Black adults have 49.6% prevalence.
https://www.cdc.gov/obesity/data/adult.html

Question 1.3

A large study including analysis of data pooled from many prospective studies showed hazard ratio (HR) and BMI relationship among non-smokers with a simplified graph shown below.

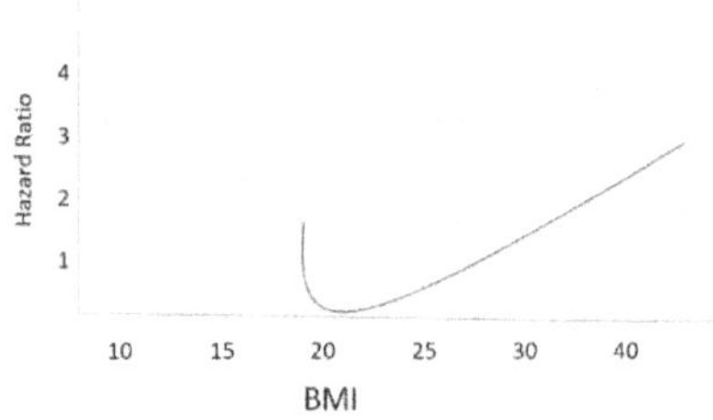

Figure (1)

Select the correct answer

a. This graph shows an "S" shaped relationship
b. The graph forms "J" shaped relationship
c. The graph does not form "S" or "J" relationship
d. The graph shows a symmetric "U" relationship

The correct answer is "b."

Question 1.4

Select the correct statement about additional information evident from this graph

a. Hazard ratio (HR) in BMI range of 25 to less than 30 is not increased

b. Hazard ratio (HR) in BMI range of 25 to less than 30 is decreased

c. There is a linear relationship between hazard ratio (HR) and BMI from BMI values 25 to 40

d. There is an inverse relationship between HR and BMI value up to around 40 BMI

The correct answer is "c."

The graph is a typical "J" shaped curve. There is a linear relationship between these two variables once BMI increases beyond 25 to 30.
Berrington de Gonzalez A. et al. N Engl J Med. 2010:363:2211-2219

Question 1.5

Prospective data in the United States shows that the relative risk of cancer-related mortality is increased in the obese population. Which of the following cancers have the highest mortality in patients with high BMI?

a. Cervical cancer
b. Uterine cancer
c. Pancreatic cancer
d. Renal cancer

The correct answer is "b."

Relative risk (RR) of mortality from cancer is higher in women as compared to men. The highest risk is for uterine cancer. It is (RR) is 6.25. It is 2.76 for pancreatic cancer, 3.20 for cervical cancer and 4.75 for renal carcinoma.
Prospective Studies Collaboration, et al, Lancet. 2009: 373:1083-1096

Question 1.6

According to the American Medical Association Expert Committee recommendations, workup of obesity in children with comorbidities should include the following:

a. Lipid profile, liver profile, blood glucose, and kidney function tests for children above the 95th percentile

b. Only lipid profile and blood glucose tests for children above the 95th percentile

c. Lipid profile, liver profile, blood glucose, and kidney function tests for children between 80 to 85th percentile

d. Lipid profile, liver profile, blood glucose, and kidney function tests for children between 75th to 80th percentile

e. Lipid profile, liver profile, blood glucose, and kidney function tests are not recommended for children above the 85th percentile

The correct answer is "a."

According to the American Medical Association Expert Committee recommendations for childhood obesity, tests mentioned in option "a." should be performed as part of workup of obese children whose BMI is more than 95th percentile. It should be noted that kidney functions are added to the profile needed for this percentile group. The yield of tests is high in patients above 95th percentile brackets.

Rao, G. Childhood obesity: highlights of AMA Expert Committee recommendations. Am Fam Physician. 2008;78:56-63.

Question 1.7

Risk factors for Obstructive Sleep Apnea include all the following except

a. Neck circumference 17 inches and more for men
b. Neck circumference 16 inches and more for women
c. Younger obese people are more likely to have obstructive sleep apnea than older ones of similar weights
d. Upper body obesity
e. An obese person with Malampati's class 3

The correct answer is "c."

Neck circumference of more than 40 cm, or 16 inches in women, and 43 cm, or 17 inches in men with upper body obesity are identified as risk factors for obstructive sleep apnea. Males are at higher risk compared to females. Similarly, older people have a higher risk of developing obstructive sleep apnea than younger ones. Malampati's anesthesia classification class 3 and above have a higher risk of presence of sleep apnea.

Flegal, K. M. (2002). Prevalence and Trends in Obesity Among US Adults, 1999-2000. Jama, 288(14), 1723-1727. doi:10.1001/jama.288.14.1723

Tucker, L. A., & Friedman, G. M. (1998). Obesity and Absenteeism: An Epidemiologic Study of 10,825 Employed Adults. American Journal of Health Promotion, 12(3), 202-207. doi:10.4278/0890-1171-12.3.202

May AL, Freedman D, Sherry B, Blanck H. Obesity - the United States, 1999-2010. MMWR Surveill Sum 2013;62(3): 120-128

Question 1.8

Which of the following medical conditions is more common in the older age group of obese women compared to obese men?

a. Diabetes Type 2
b. Osteoarthrosis of the knees
c. Obstructive Sleep Apnea
d. Alzheimer's Disease

The correct answer is "d."

In later life, obesity seems to be associated with an increased risk of development of Alzheimer's dementia. This association appears stronger in women.

Gustafson, D., Rothenberg, E., Blennow, K., Steen, B., & Skoog, I. (2003). An 18-Year Follow-up of Overweight and Risk of Alzheimer Disease. Archives of Internal Medicine, 163(13), 1524-1528. doi:10.1001/archinte.163.13.1524

Question 1.9

Which class of obesity is assigned to a patient with BMI of 37?

a. Overweight
b. Class I obesity
c. Class II obesity
d. Class III obesity

The correct answer is "c."

Healthy BMI falls in range 18.5 to 24.9. Overweight is 25 to 29.9. Class I falls in the range of 30.0 to 34.9. Class II is 35 to 39.9. Class III has BMI value of more than 40. WHO classifies weight categories into six groups starting from under-weight for less than 18.5 to categories as stated above. BMI of 50 or above is considered as super morbid obesity according to some published surgical literature.

The SuRF Report 2 (PDF). The Surveillance of Risk Factors Report Series (SuRF). World Health Organization. 2005. p. 22.

Question 1.10

A husband and wife are seen in their family doctor's office. Height and weight are measured for both. Body composition reports are generated using a proprietary body fat analyzer. The reports show that body fat percentages are 17 and 33 percent for husband and wife respectively. Please select the correct statement.

a. Husband is likely to be an athlete

b. Husband is obese

c. Wife has an acceptable value of the fat composition

d. Wife has Obesity

The correct answer is "d."

Based on expert opinion, the following percentage body fat numbers have been suggested. These figures are, however, yet to be validated scientifically. Women who are ≥ 32% and men ≥ 25% fall in the range of obesity. 25 - 31% for women and 18 to 24% for men are acceptable numbers. Fitness range is 21 to 24 % for women and 14 to 17% for men. Athletes can have 14-20% and 6 - 13% for women and men, respectively.

Author Natalie Digate Muth Health and Fitness Expert Natalie Digate Muth. "What Are the Guidelines for Percentage of Body Fat Loss?" ACE, www.acefitness.org/acefit/healthy-living-article/60/112/what-are-the-guidelines-for-percentage-of-body-fat.

Question 1.11

A 25-year-old male with a BMI of 40 is following a Bariatric program. He is recently diagnosed with sleep apnea and insulin resistance. It is a wakeup call for him. He makes dramatic changes in lifestyle. He indulges in heavy resistance exercises and goes to the gym, almost daily. He feels that he is losing inches but not much weight. In the follow-up visit, he is counseled about the possible reasons and how to better evaluate the resolution of obesity. Which of the following statements is most appropriate?

a. BMI remains as the best way to track his progress in future months
b. BMI is more useful than % body fat (BF) to see his progress
c. A more helpful tool may be % body fat
d. % Body fat is not a very useful tool in this situation to monitor his progress

The correct answer is "c."

% BF is considered as a more accurate tool when a significant increase in muscle mass is anticipated.

Question 1.12

Which of the racial descents have higher risk for cardiovascular disease, diabetes type 2, and development of metabolic syndrome?

a. Japanese
b. Native Americans
c. South Asians
d. Scandinavians

The correct answer is "c."

People of South Asian descent have shown features of insulin resistance, higher lipid levels, more visceral fat, higher leptin levels, and high inflammatory cytokine levels as compared to other nations. For the same reasons, their obesity criteria cut-offs have lower thresholds.

Holland, Ariel T., et al. “Spectrum of Cardiovascular Diseases in Asian-American Racial/Ethnic Subgroups.” Annals of Epidemiology, vol. 21, no. 8, 2011, pp. 608–614., doi:10.1016/j.annepidem.2011.04.004.

Etiology

Question 2.1

Which of the followings is the correct statement about etiology of obesity in the American population?

a. Substantial portion sizes
b. The increased popularity of Fast Food.
c. High energy but the lower nutrient density of food.
d. Low cost of processed food
e. All the above statements are correct

The correct answer is "e."

Statements “a.” to “d.” all hold true in the development of obesity in United States. Substantial portion sizes with consumption of energy-rich diets along with a low cost of processed foods is contributing to the problem of obesity.

Levian C, Ruiz E, Yang X. The pathogenesis of obesity from a genomic and systems biology perspective. Yale J Biol Med 2014; 87(2): 113–126

Question 2.2

Which of the following statements is true regarding the prevalence of obesity?

a. In the United States, the prevalence of obesity is more in higher socioeconomic segments of the population

b. In the United States, the prevalence of obesity is equal in both higher and lower socioeconomic segments of the population

c. In the United States, the prevalence of obesity is more in lower socioeconomic segments of the population

d. In developing countries, the prevalence of obesity is similar to the distribution of obesity seen in the United States

e. In developing countries, the prevalence of obesity is more in lower socioeconomic groups

The correct answer is "c."

This fact reflects the specific challenges to lower socioeconomic groups where education, access to healthcare, and other resources are less as compared to more affluent segments of society.

Tillotson, J. E. (2004). AMERICAS OBESITY: Conflicting Public Policies, Industrial Economic Development, and Unintended Human Consequences. Annual Review of Nutrition, 24(1), 617-643. doi: 10.1146/annurev.nutr.24.012003.132434

Question 2.3

It is established that certain prenatal factors may increase the risk of developing obesity in later life. Which of the following statements is true?

a. Maternal malnutrition and diabetes can predispose an individual to develop diabetes and obesity in later life
b. Low birth weight babies whose mothers have malnutrition in the first two trimesters are more prone to develop obesity in later life.
c. Smoking during pregnancy by mothers can increase the risk of obesity by several folds
d. Breastfed babies are less prone to develop obesity as compared to bottle-fed infants.
e. All above statements are correct

The correct answer is "e."

In recent years, several events related to the prenatal developmental phase and subsequent development of obesity have been recognized. Maternal malnutrition, diabetes, and smoking have been suggested as contributing factors for adulthood obesity. Historically, breastfeeding seemed to have a beneficial effect, but some studies appear to challenge this.

Lillycrop, K. A., & Burdge, G. C. (2010). Epigenetic changes in early life and future risk of obesity. International Journal of Obesity, 35(1), 72-83. doi:10.1038/ijo.2010.122

Question 2.4

Which of the following genotype is related to the most common type of monogenic obesity?

a. Lipase hormone sensitive (LIPE) gene
b. Glucocorticoid receptor (NCR3C1) gene
c. G protein beta3 subunit (GNß3)
d. Melanocortin 4 receptor (MCR4) gene
e. Uncoupling protein 3 (UCP3)

The correct answer is "d."

Melanocortin 4 receptor deficiency runs in affected families. Salient features include early childhood obesity and hyperphagia. Metabolic workup shows insulin resistance, increased bone mineral density, and greater than expected linear growth. Gene polymorphism located at chromosome 18q22 is suggested.

Shriner D, et al. Genetic contributions to the development of obesity. In: Akabas S, Lederman S, Moore B, eds. Textbook of Obesity: Biological, Psychological, and Cultural Influences. West Sussex, UK: Wiley-Blackwell; 2012, pp. 79-86

Bays H, Scinta W: Adiposopathy and epigenetics: an introduction to obesity as a transgenerational disease. Curr Med Res Opin 2015 31:2059-2069.

10.1185/03007995.2015.1087983
https://www.ncbi.nlm.nih.gov/pubmed/26331354

Chung WK: An overview of monogenic and syndromic obesities in humans. Pediatr Blood Cancer 2012 58:122-128. 10.1002/pbc.23372
https://www.ncbi.nlm.nih.gov/pubmed/21994130

Question 2.5

Single gene mutations can lead to monogenic obesity. Select the correct answer regarding monogenic obesity.

a. It is the most common form of obesity
b. It manifests in adult life
c. Affected genes belong primarily to the function of leptin-melanocortin pathways
d. Features of this kind of obesity include early onset, extreme obesity, increased food intake, and energy storage
e. “c.” and “d.” are correct

The correct answer is "e."

Monogenic obesity is uncommon and is seen in early life. Affected subjects are extremely obese. More than 1500 related genes have been reported; examples include genes for Leptin (LEP), Leptin receptor (LEPR), Proopiomelanocortin (POMC), Melanocortin 4 receptor (MC4R).

Yale J, Levian C, Ruiz E, Yang X. The pathogenesis of obesity from a genomic and systems biology perspective. Biol Med 2014;87(2):113-26. eCollection 2014

Question 2.6

Which of the followings is the most common human obesity syndrome?

a. Bardet-Biedl syndrome
b. Wilson-Turner syndrome
c. Cohen syndrome
d. Prader-Willi syndrome
e. Börjeson-Forssman-Lehmann syndrome

The correct answer is "d."

Prader-Willi Syndrome is the most common syndromic obesity in humans. Its features include progressive weight gain, decreased fetal activity, hypotonia, mental retardation, short stature, small hands and feet, hypogonadism, and hyperphagia between the first and second years of life.

Pérusse, L., Chagnon, Y. C., & Bouchard, C. (1998). Etiology of Massive Obesity: Role of Genetic Factors. World Journal of Surgery, 22(9), 907-912. doi:10.1007/s002689900493

Question 2.7

Regarding MC4R (Melanocortin 4 receptor) deficiency, which of the following statements is not correct?

a. Heterozygous mutation is the most common monogenic form of obesity in childhood

b. It is associated with early-onset obesity

c. It is associated with shorter than average height

d. Fasting insulin levels are high in patients with MC4R deficiency

The correct answer is "c."

Congenital deficiency of MC4R gene features obesity in both childhood and adult life. The onset of obesity is early and these patients are taller. High insulin levels may be contributory to the growth acceleration.

Savastano, D. M., Tanofsky-Kraff, M., Han, J. C., Ning, C., Sorg, R. A., Roza, C. A., . . . Yanovski, J. A. (2009). Energy intake and energy expenditure among children with polymorphisms of the melanocortin-3 receptor. American Journal of Clinical Nutrition, 90(4), 912-920. doi:10.3945/ajcn.2009.27537

Question 2.8

Which of the following syndromes is characterized by progressive obesity, diminished fetal activity, hypotonia after birth, mental retardation, short stature, behavioral abnormalities, hypogonadism, small hands, and feet, and hyperphagia?

a. Bardet-Biedl syndrome
b. Wilson-Turner syndrome
c. Cohen syndrome
d. Prader-Willi syndrome
e. Börjeson-Forssman-Lehmann syndrome

The correct answer is "d."

Prader-Willi Syndrome is associated with hypotonia, stunted growth, mental retardation, short height, hypogonadism, hyperphagia, small hands and feet, and behavioral issues.

Question 2.9

Which of the following syndromes is characterized by polydactyly, developmental delay, impairment of vision, hypogonadism, central obesity, and renal abnormalities?

a. Bardet-Biedl syndrome

b. Wilson-Turner syndrome

c. Cohen syndrome

d. Prader-Willi syndrome

e. Börjeson-Forssman-Lehmann Syndrome

The correct answer is "a."

Bardet-Biedl syndrome results from an autosomal recessive gene mutation (BBS genes). Ciliary action of cells is affected. Defects in smell, vision, and hearing are seen in addition to abnormalities of chemical signals and cell movements.

Forsythe, Elizabeth, and Philip L Beales. "Bardet–Biedl Syndrome." European Journal of Human Genetics, vol. 21, no. 1, 2012, pp. 8–13., doi:10.1038/ejhg.2012.115.

Question 2.10

Select the correct statement regarding Gourmand syndrome.

a. Etiology is damage to the right frontal lobe
b. The mechanism includes the loss of downstream satiety signaling from the hypothalamus
c. These patients develop a new, post-injury passion for gourmet food
d. All the above statements are correct

The correct answer is "d."

This eating disorder is seen in persons with affected right anterior cerebral hemispheric areas. In addition to eating other impulse control disorders may be present. Abnormalities of the serotonergic system have been proposed as well.

Regard, M., and Landis, T., "'Gourmand Syndrome': Eating Passion Associated with Right Anterior Lesions." Neurology, vol. 48, no. 5, Jan. 1997, pp. 1185–1190., doi:10.1212/wnl.48.5.1185.

Question 2.11

WAGR Obesity Syndrome is characterized by which of the following features?

a. Wilms tumor
b. Aniridia
c. Genitourinary anomalies
d. Mental retardation and obesity
e. All the above

The correct answer is "e."

This syndrome involves a deletion mutation on chromosome 11 (11p13 region). Patients are predisposed to risk of developing Wilms tumor. Other features include abnormalities of the reproductive and urinary tracts. Intellectual disabilities are also seen.

Turleau, C., Grouchy, J. D., Nihoul-Fékété, C., Dufier, J. L., Chavin-Colin, F., & Junien, C. (1984). Del11p13/nephroblastoma without aniridia. Human Genetics, 67(4), 455-456. doi:10.1007/bf00291410

Question 2.12

Regarding craniopharyngiomas, all the following are true EXCEPT

a. It is a rare hypothalamic tumor that leads to obesity
b. It is characterized by peak incidence rates at ages 5-15 and 50-60 years
c. Hyperinsulinemia and leptin resistance is seen in these patients
d. Reduced sympathetic tone leads to low physical activity and low metabolic rate
e. Surgical resection of the hypothalamus is mostly curative

The correct answer is "e."

Statements “a.,” “b., “c.,” and “d.” are correct. Surgery is not always curative. Tumor recurrence is high in the initial years. In instances of subtotal removal, 5-year disease free rate is 48.3%.

“Craniopharyngioma.” Wikipedia, Wikimedia Foundation, 11 Aug. 2018, en.wikipedia.org/wiki/Craniopharyngioma.

Question 2.13

A hormone has the following characteristics

1. Its level increases during diet induced weight loss
2. Its level increases with sleep deprivation
3. It mediates the sense of hunger
4. IV administration decreases fat oxidation and increases food intake with adiposity

Which of the following hormones has the features stated above?

a. Ghrelin

b. Leptin

c. Testosterone

d. Thyroid hormone

e. Growth hormone

The correct answer is "a."

Ghrelin is a peptide hormone which is produced by the GI tract. It is one of the neuropeptides regulating appetite and energy homeostasis.

Kojima, M., Hosoda, H., Date, Y., Nakazato, M., Matsuo, H., & Kangawa, K. (1999). Ghrelin is a growth-hormone-releasing acylated peptide from stomach. Nature, 402(6762), 656-660. doi:10.1038/45230

Question 2.14

Regarding CNS regulation of hunger, all the following are anorexigens (inhibitors of hunger) EXCEPT

a. POMC (proopiomelanocortin)
b. α-MSH (α-Melanocyte-stimulating hormone)
c. CART (cocaine-and amphetamine-regulated transcript)
d. NPY (neuropeptide Y)

The correct answer is "d."

Neuropeptide Y is a neuropeptide in the mammalian nervous system. Its promotes food intake and storage of fat. Additionally, it helps control anxiety, stress, and pain. All other options stated above have anorexigenic effects.

Decressac, M., & Barker, R. (2012). Neuropeptide Y and its role in CNS disease and repair. Experimental Neurology, 238(2), 265-272. doi: 10.1016/j.expneurol.2012.09.004

Question 2.15

All the following neurohormones are orexigens (stimulators of hunger) EXCEPT

a. NPY (Neuropeptide Y)
b. Agouti Related Peptide (AgRP)
c. Serotonin
d. MCH (Melanin-concentrating hormone)

The correct answer is "c."

Serotonin is an appetite suppressant. More than 80 percent of the body's serotonin is produced in GI tract. Serotonin is also produced in the brain. It does affect mood and emotional energy. It is known that the consumption of carbohydrates before meals can suppress hunger and lead to less overall consumption of food.

Question 2.16

Neuropeptide Y (NPY) plays a significant role in hunger and weight maintenance. Select the correct statement regarding this hormone.

a. It increases food intake (orexigenic)
b. It promotes storage of fat

c. Stimulated by Ghrelin

d. In obese patients elevated levels of NPY are seen

e. All the above statements are correct

The correct answer is "e."

NPY is a neuropeptide which consists of 36 amino acids. High concentrations are seen in hypothalamus, hippocampus and acuate nucleus. It promotes food intake, fat storage and promotes cell growth.

Schwartz, M. W. (1992). Inhibition of hypothalamic neuropeptide Y gene expression by insulin. Endocrinology, 130(6), 3608-3616. doi:10.1210/en.130.6.3608

Question 2.17

Regarding AgRP (Agouti Related Peptide), which of the following statements is not correct?

a. It is an orexigenic chemical

b. Found in first-order neurons in arcuate nucleus

c. Keeps hunger from turning down.

d. Acts on MC3R and MC4R receptors on second-order neurons to block effects of ROMC/CART (α-MSH)

e. It is primarily an anorexigenic hormone

The correct answer is "e."

Agouti-related protein (AgRP) is closely related to neuropeptide Y (NPY) as both neuropeptides are produced by the same cells in the hypothalamus. This neuropeptide is orexigenic. It is thought to cause obesity by chronic inhibition of MC4-R. This peptide possibly has a role in stress-related eating issues and eating disorders.

Jackson, P.J. et al. (2006) Structural and molecular evolutionary analysis of Agouti and Agouti-related proteins. Chem. Biol. 13, 1297–1305

Question 2.18

Orexin and MCH (melanocyte-concentrating hormone) are neurohormones. All the following statements are correct EXCEPT

a. These are orexigenic chemicals
b. Found in second-order neurons in the lateral hypothalamus
c. These hormones are anorexigenic
d. They act on higher order neurons to stimulate arousal, anxiety, aggression, feeding, pleasure, reward, and learning

The correct answer is "c."

Orexin and MCH both have a role in sleep regulation and are considered to be orexigenic.

Delgado, J.M. and Anand, B.K. (1953) "Increase of food intake induced by electrical stimulation of the lateral hypothalamus," The American Journal of Physiology. 172 (1): 162–168.

Question 2.19

Which of the following statements is not correct regarding proopiomelanocortin (POMC)?

a. It is an anorexigenic hormone
b. It is found in first-order neurons in arcuate nucleus
c. It releases α- MSH which acts on second-order neuron MC3R and MC4R receptors.
d. It is orexigenic in nature

The correct answer is "d."

The pituitary gland produces POMC. It has anorexigenic properties and acts on melanocortin 4 receptors.

Question 2.20

Which of the following statements is not correct regarding cocaine-and amphetamine-regulated transcript (CART)?

a. It is anorexigenic in nature
b. It is found with NPY in arcuate nucleus or alone in lateral hypothalamus

c. Its mechanism of action may involve the central release of GLP-1

d. It is orexigenic in nature

The correct answer is "d."

CART hypoactivity in the hypothalamus causes hyperphagia and weight gain in experimental animals.

Nakhate, K. T., Kokare, D. M., Singru, P. S., & Subhedar, N. K. (2010). Central regulation of feeding behavior during social isolation of rat: evidence for the role of endogenous CART system. International Journal of Obesity, 35(6), 773-784. doi:10.1038/ijo.2010.231

Question 2.21

Select the correct statement regarding leptin.

a. It is an anorexigenic in nature

b. It is primarily produced by white adipose tissue

c. Its mechanism of action involves direct stimulation of POMC/CART, turns off GABA inhibition of POMC and inhibits orexin.

d. Its mechanism of action involves inhibition of NPY/AgRP

e. All above statements are correct

The correct answer is "e."

White adipose tissue produces leptin. It has a role in glucose homeostasis, reproduction, inflammation, and energy homeostasis. Leptin levels are increased in obesity.

Question 2.22

Select the incorrect statement regarding leptin deficiency.

a. It is the most common form of obesity in humans
b. Affected individuals are affected in early childhood
c. Leptin levels are high in patients with leptin receptor defects
d. Puberty is delayed and hypogonadism is seen in affected individuals

The correct answer is "a."

Congenital leptin deficiency related to obesity is an extremely rare disorder. Leptin has not been useful in treating common and complex obesity.

Kelesidis, T. (2010). Narrative Review: The Role of Leptin in Human Physiology: Emerging Clinical Applications. Annals of Internal Medicine, 152(2), 93-100. doi:10.7326/0003-4819-152-2-201001190-00008

Question 2.23

Which of the following statements is true?

a. Testosterone levels and insulin resistance has an inverse relationship

b. PPAR-α (peroxisome proliferator-activated receptor alpha) is active under conditions of excess energy

c. Growth hormone deficiency increases lean body mass

d. Hyperthyroidism may cause fluid retention, decreased metabolism, and weight gain

e. Growth hormone excess increases visceral fat mass

The correct answer is "a."

Testosterone levels and insulin resistance share an inverse relationship with each other. Growth hormone leads to increased lean body mass. Hypothyroidism can cause fluid retention and weight gain. Growth hormone causes a decrease in visceral fat mass. PPAR-α is active in situations of energy deprivation.

Question 2.24

A young female presents with central obesity, insulin resistance, hyperinsulinemia, diabetes, and excessive hair growth on the face. Select the correct statement.

a. This patient is unlikely to have infertility
b. Insulin level is likely to be low
c. Lipoprotein lipase is expected to be more active
d. Menstrual periods are expected to be unaffected
e. Metformin is contraindicated in these cases

The correct answer is "c."

Features mentioned above represent a typical case of the polycystic ovarian syndrome. Infertility, high insulin levels and abnormalities of menstrual cycles are commonly observed. Metformin is one of the widely prescribed medications for this disorder. Lipoprotein lipase is a fat storage enzyme. It leads to more visceral fat deposition. In younger girls after menarche, cyclic menstrual abnormalities may be seen. The initial period of observation without specific treatment may be appropriate.

Jensen MD. Obesity. In: Goldman L, Schafer A, eds. Cecil Textbook of Medicine, 24th ed. Philadelphia, PA: Saunders Elsevier; 2012, pp. 1409-17.

Question 2.25

A hormone has the following features.

1. It is derived from fat
2. It is anorexigenic
3. It reduces food intake
4. Its levels are increased in obesity

Which of the following hormones is discussed above?

a. Ghrelin
b. Testosterone
c. Growth hormone
d. Leptin
e. Insulin

The correct answer is "d."

Leptin is the hormone with features stated above.

O'rourke, R. W. (2014). Metabolic Thrift and the Genetic Basis of Human Obesity. Annals of Surgery, 259(4), 642-648. doi:10.1097/sla.0000000000000361

Question 2.26

Which of the following statements is correct regarding adipocytes?

a. Lipoprotein lipase is involved in fat elaboration and released from adipocytes
b. Hormone-sensitive lipase is involved in storing fat
c. Adiponectin is the most abundant adipokine in fat
d. Adiponectin levels are increased during obesity
e. Adipocytes do not play a significant role in the outcomes of obesity

The correct answer is "c."

Adiponectin is the most abundant adipokine in fat cells. It leads to increased insulin sensitivity and decreases changes induced by tumor necrosis factor-alpha (TNF-α). Lipoprotein lipase is involved in the storage of fat. Hormone-sensitive lipase, on the other hand, is involved in elaboration and release of fat from adipocytes.

Racette SB, Deusinger SS, Deusinger RH. Obesity: Overview of prevalence, etiology, and treatment. Phys Ther. 2003;83(3): 276-88

Question 2.27

Which of the following statements is correct regarding the influence of psychological factors in the development of obesity?

a. Restraint disinhibition may be a critical factor in the etiology of obesity

b. History of sexual abuse during childhood can lead to the development of obesity in later life

c. Binge eating disorder involves the consumption of a significant amount of food in 2 hours period characterized by a feeling of loss of control. It is estimated in up to 50% cases who seek bariatric surgery

d. Night eating disorder involves the consumption of up to 25% of one's daily caloric intake during the evening and night. It happens at least two times per week for at least three months

e. All above are correct

The correct answer is "e."

Here choices "a," to "d." are all correct. It is recognized that restraint disinhibition, history of sexual abuse in childhood, binge eating, and night eating disorders contribute to the development of obesity.

In binge eating disorder patients consume a large quantity of food more than once every week for the last three months. It is identified in 2-3 percent of the adult population in the United States. More than half of patients with severe obesity are thought to have this eating disorder. Patients do not show behaviors like purging or excessive exercise. Lisdexamfetamine has been found to be useful in the treatment of this disorder. This medicine is a Schedule II drug. This drug has the potential for abuse and dependence.

Redinger, R. N. (2008). The Prevalence and Etiology of Nongenetic Obesity and Associated Disorders. Southern Medical Journal, 101(4), 395-399. doi: 10.1097/01.smj.0000308879.67271.09nia

Question 2.28

Which of the following statements is true for the etiology of development of obesity?

a. Overweight individuals have low levels of C-reactive proteins

b. Different microorganisms have been studied as possible etiologies of obesity. Avian adenovirus SMAM-1 and human adenovirus Ad-36 have been suspected to have a link to develop obesity

c. The gut microbiome is not linked to the development of obesity

d. Majority of children who tested positive for Ad-36 are not likely to be obese

e. All above are correct

The correct answer is "b."

C-reactive protein levels are raised in obese individuals. There is evidence that gut microbiome is linked to the development of obesity. Several viruses are suspected to have some link with the development of obesity.

Atkinson, R. L. (2007). Viruses as an Etiology of Obesity. Mayo Clinic Proceedings, 82(10), 1192-1198.
doi:10.4065/82.10.1192

Question 2.29

Which of the following statements is true regarding eating behaviors?

a. Having a regular breakfast routine may help prevent obesity
b. People consuming more than 33% of the daily intake of energy in the evening are twice more likely to have obesity
c. Fat storage tendency of the body is increased during late evening hours
d. Caffeine, ethanol, and sodium may alter circadian rhythms and can have a possible role in the development of obesity
e. All the above statements are correct

The correct answer is "e."

Regular breakfast seems to help prevent weight gain. Late night eating is a risk factor to develop obesity as the dynamics of various hormones change during the night. Similarly, excessive caffeine and alcohol consumption may also contribute to the weight gain.

Question 2.30

Which of the following statements is true regarding eating behaviors?

a. High calcium in the diet increases the risk of gaining weight by inhibiting metabolic pathways
b. Fast eaters are less likely to be obese
c. Consumption of some vitamins like niacin and vitamin C can promote obesity
d. Regularly consuming food high in protein and fat, like cheese, cannot be a significant factor in the development of obesity
e. None of the above statements is true

The correct answer is "c."

The stimulant effect of niacin (B3) has been reported. Similarly, high doses of B1 and B2 are linked to the development of obesity. Vitamin C can adversely affect reactive oxygen element level to cause weight gain. Consumption of copious amounts of full-fat cheese can contribute to weight gain too.

Zhou, S. (2014). Excess vitamin intake: An unrecognized risk factor for obesity. World J Diabetes, 5(1), 1. doi:10.4239/wjd.v5.i1.1

Question 2.31

Which of the following statements regarding the consumption of sugar in liquid form compared to solid form is correct?

a. Gastric emptying and transit time increases

b. Reduced postprandial ghrelin suppression

c. Increased postprandial hunger

d. Larger calorie intake in subsequent meals

e. All above statements are correct

The correct answer is "e."

The effects of liquid sugars include increased emptying of the stomach, less suppression of postprandial ghrelin, and increased post-meal hunger with increased consumption in following meals.

Dimeglio, D., & Mattes, R. (2000). Liquid versus solid carbohydrate: effects on food intake and body weight. International Journal of Obesity, 24(6), 794-800. doi: 10.1038/sj.ijo.0801229

Question 2.32

Resting energy expenditure and non-exercise activity thermogenesis have an essential role in the health and development of obesity. Which of the following statements is true?

a. Resting energy expenditure is 15 to 20% of daily energy expenditure

b. People living in Arctic areas are more likely to have a low BMR (basal metabolic rate)

c. BMR is inversely proportional to lean body mass

d. An extra hour of being seated daily than just standing may lead to around 6 pounds of weight gain a year

e. Energy-restricted diets are unlikely to change BMI

The correct answer is "d."

A fair amount of evidence exists to prove the ill effects of sedentary lifestyles. Resting energy expenditure is typically 60 to 70% of total energy expenditure. People with higher lean body mass are expected to have higher BMR. Cold weather may lead to more burning of calories.

Weinsier, RL, Hunter, GR, Heini, AF, Goran, MI, Sell, SM. (1998) The etiology of obesity relative contribution of metabolic factors, diet, and physical activity. Am J Med. 105(2),145-50.

Question 2.33

Which of the following statements is true regarding Thermic Effect of Food (TEF), Non-Exercise Activity Thermogenesis (NEAT) and Physical Activity (PA)?

a. Approximately 20% of TEF is obligatory (digestion, absorption, and storage of nutrients) and 80 % is facultative thermogenesis
b. TEF is higher in insulin-resistant obese individuals
c. Lower levels of NEAT may predict future weight gain
d. Epidemiologically, the role of PA in obesity and weight gain is less consistent than the role of energy intake to the development of obesity
e. None of the above statements is true

The correct answer is "c."

60 to 70 % of the thermic effect of meals is obligatory, and the remaining 30 to 40 % is facultative thermogenesis. Lower levels of NEAT can contribute to weight gain.

Tappy, L. (1996). Thermic effect of food and sympathetic nervous system activity in humans. Reproduction Nutrition Development, 36(4), 391-397. doi:10.1051/rnd:19960405

Weinsier, RL, Hunter, GR, Heini, AF, Goran, MI, Sell, SM. (1998) The etiology of obesity relative contribution of metabolic factors, diet, and physical activity. Am J Med. 105(2),145-50.

Question 2.34

Energy homeostasis is essential in the maintenance of weight. It has various components. Two of the important ones are "Basal Metabolic Rate" (BMR) and "Physical Activity" (PA). Which of the following statements is correct?

a. Basal metabolic rate constitutes approximately 20 to 30% of total body expenditure of energy
b. Basal metabolic rate constitutes approximately 60 to 70 % of total body expenditure of energy
c. Physical activity accounts 60 to 70% of total body expenditure of energy.
d. Physical activity accounts for 40 to 50% of total body expenditure of energy.

The correct answer is "b."

60 to 70 percent of body energy is spent by BMR. Physical activity is among one of the most modifiable factors.

Question 2.35

A 22-year-old female presents with the problem of obesity. She has a BMI of 38. Her height is about 55 inches (140 cm). She has rounded face. Oral examination shows poorly developed teeth. Some deformities of her hand and feet are noted. X-ray of hands show short fourth metacarpals in addition to deformities of other short bones. She has a calcium level of 6.6 mg/dl. Phosphate is low. A genetic cause is suspected. Please select the correct diagnosis.

a. Prader-Willi syndrome
b. Albright's hereditary osteodystrophy
c. Cohen syndrome
d. Down's syndrome

The correct answer is "b."

Features mentioned in the problem suggest Albright's hereditary osteodystrophy. It is a G protein abnormality due to the defective gene (GNAS1). On the other hand, Cohen syndrome is due to an autosomal recessive gene mutation at VPS13B (COH1 gene). It is associated with developmental delay, retinal abnormalities, thick eyebrows, and eyelashes, hypotonia, laxity of ligaments, low IQ, and smaller head size.

Bays H, Scinta W: Adiposopathy and epigenetics: an introduction to obesity as a transgenerational disease. Curr Med Res Opin 2015 31:2059-2069. 10.1185/03007995.2015.1087983 https://www.ncbi.nlm.nih.gov/pubmed/26331354

Obesity – Relation with Other Diseases

Question 3.1

Which of the following statements regarding the relation of obesity to other diseases is correct?

a. Higher incidence of cancer-related mortality exists in obese patients with cancers of colon, rectum, gallbladder, liver, pancreas, kidney, esophagus, myelomas, and some of the lymphomas

b. Osteoarthrosis risk increases by three folds in people with BMI more than 27

c. Non-alcoholic fatty liver disease (NAFLD) may affect up to 70 percent of patients with type 2 diabetes mellitus

d. Prevalence of major depression increases to almost four times once BMI exceeds from 25 to 35

e. All the above statements are correct

The correct answer is "e."

The incidence of various cancers and related mortality is higher in the obese population. Other disorders like osteoarthrosis, fatty liver disease, and depression also occur at an increased frequency.

Wright, M. E., Chang, S., Schatzkin, A., Albanes, D., Kipnis, V., Mouw, T., . . . Leitzmann, M. F. (2007). Prospective study of adiposity and weight change in relation to prostate cancer incidence and mortality. Cancer, 109(4), 675-684. doi:10.1002/cncr.22443

Reijman, M., Pols, H. A., Bergink, A. P., Hazes, J. M., Belo, J. N., Lievense, A. M., & Bierma-Zeinstra, S. M. (2006). Body mass index associated with onset and progression of osteoarthritis of the knee but not of the hip: The Rotterdam Study. Annals of the Rheumatic Diseases, 66(2), 158-162. doi:10.1136/ard.2006.053538

Adams, L. A. (2006). Treatment of non-alcoholic fatty liver disease. Postgraduate Medical Journal, 82(967), 315-322. doi:10.1136/pgmj.2005.042200

Question 3.2

Which of the following statements about the relation between obesity and sleep apnea is correct?

a. Apnea-hypopnea index is likely to increase with an increase in BMI

b. Apnea-hypopnea index is likely to decrease with an increase in BMI

c. Apnea-hypopnea index is unlikely to decrease with a decrease in BMI

d. Apnea-hypopnea index has an inverse relation with a change in BMI

e. None of the above statements are correct

The correct answer is "a."

Increasing BMI has a close association with the development of obstructive sleep apnea. It may also worsen the pre-existing condition. Apnea-hypopnea index is a ratio to determine the severity of sleep apnea.

Schmid, S. M., Hallschmid, M., & Schultes, B. (2015). The metabolic burden of sleep loss. The Lancet Diabetes & Endocrinology, 3(1), 52-62. doi:10.1016/s2213-8587(14)70012-9

Question 3.3

Obesity is known to have a paradoxical effect on which one of the following conditions?

a. Diabetes type 2
b. Essential hypertension
c. Obstructive sleep apnea
d. Congestive heart failure (CHF)
e. Arthritis

The correct answer is "d."

Paradoxical effect on CHF is sometimes noted with obesity. It is observed that weight loss may worsen CHF in some cases.

Kenchaiah, S., Evans, J. C., Levy, D., Wilson, P. W., Benjamin, E. J., Larson, M. G., . . . Vasan, R. S. (2002). Obesity and the Risk of Heart Failure. New England Journal of Medicine, 347(5), 305-313. doi:10.1056/nejmoa020245

Question 3.4

Weight loss is unlikely to improve which of the following conditions?

a. Diabetes type 2

b. Obstructive sleep apnea

c. Osteoporosis

d. Risk of multi-organ cancer

e. Fatty liver

The correct answer is "c."

All the conditions stated above are likely to improve with losing weight, except osteoporosis. It is risk remains unchanged in most cases.

Shapses, Sue A., and Deeptha Sukumar. Annual Review of Nutrition, U.S. National Library of Medicine, 21 Aug. 2012, www.ncbi.nlm.nih.gov/pmc/articles/PMC4016236/.

Question 3.5

Various cancers are more common in the obese population. The risk of which of the following cancer types does <u>not</u> increase with increasing BMI?

a. Breast cancer

b. Colon cancer

c. Endometrial cancer

d. Lung cancer

e. Pancreas

The correct answer is "d."

All cancers stated above have increased risk in obese patients, except lung cancer.

Question 3.6

Adipose tissues are known to produce both pro-inflammatory and anti-inflammatory elements. Which of the following statements may hold true for an obese individual?

a. Increased tumor necrosis factor-α and interlukin-6

b. Decreased tumor necrosis factor-α, interleukin-6, leptin, and plasminogen activator inhibitor

c. Increased adiponectin, interleukin 4-10, and interlukin-1 receptor antagonist

d. Decreased leptin and plasminogen activator inhibitor

e. Increased interleukin-1 receptor antagonist

The correct answer is "a."

In obese individuals, increased levels of inflammatory cytokines are seen. Tumor necrosis factor-α and interleukin-6 levels are increased.

Odegaard, J. I., & Chawla, A. (2013). Pleiotropic Actions of Insulin Resistance and Inflammation in Metabolic Homeostasis. Science, 339(6116), 172-177. doi:10.1126/science.1230721

Question 3.7

A link between diabetes and obesity is well established. Which of the following statements is not correct regarding this link?

a. Above 80% of people with diabetes are obese. They have android morphology and raised waist to hip ratios

b. Insulin resistance leads to more visceral fat accumulation

c. Even 5 to 10% weight loss can help bring glycemic control

d. Diabetic medications such as incretin mimetics (e.g., exenatide) are likely to cause weight loss

e. Sulfonylureas and thiazolidinediones are likely to cause weight loss

The correct answer is "e."

Sulfonylureas (Amaryl®, Glucotrol®, diabeta®) and thiazolidinediones (Actos®, Avandia®) are known to cause potential weight gain. Statements "a." to "d." are correct.

Hevener, A. L., & Febbraio, M. A. (2010). The 2009 Stock Conference Report: Inflammation, Obesity, and Metabolic

Disease. Obesity Reviews, 11(9), 635-644. doi:10.1111/j.1467-789x.2009. 00691.x

*Amaryl® and diabeta® are registered trademarks of Sanofi-aventis U.S. LLC, Glucotrol® is a registered trademark of Pfizer Inc., Actos® is a registered trademark of Takeda Pharmaceutical Company, Avandia® is a registered trademark of GlaxoSmithKline plc.

Question 3.8

Regarding obesity and cardiovascular disease, which of the following statements is true?

a. The risk of cardiovascular disease in obese, diabetic women and men is 78.8% and 86.9% respectively
b. High BMI patients who present with CHF have a lower risk of hospitalization and death as compared to similar patients with normal BMI
c. Anorectic medications may be used with great precaution in patients with significant cardiovascular disease
d. Weight gain with BMI increasing from below 25 to above 30, is associated with the prevalence of HTN increasing from 15% to 40%
e. All the above statements are correct.

The correct answer is "e."

Statements "a." to "d." are all correct. This question discusses the high cardiovascular risks in obese patients. There seems to be the paradoxical effect of obesity on congestive heart failure.

Wilson, P. W., Dagostino, R. B., Sullivan, L., Parise, H., & Kannel, W. B. (2002). Overweight and Obesity as Determinants of Cardiovascular Risk. Archives of Internal Medicine, 162(16), 1867. doi:10.1001/archinte.162.16.1867

Question 3.9

Which of the following is <u>not</u> the component of diagnostic criteria for metabolic syndrome?

a. Abdominal waist circumference
b. Triglycerides and fasting blood sugar
c. High-density lipoprotein
d. Blood pressure
e. Liver function tests

The correct answer is "e."

Liver function abnormality is not included in diagnostic criteria of metabolic syndrome. All other facts stated in statements "a." to "d." are included.

Phelan, S., Wadden, T. A., Berkowitz, R. I., Sarwer, D. B., Womble, L. G., Cato, R. K., & Rothman, R. (2007). Impact of weight loss on the metabolic syndrome. International Journal of Obesity, 31(9), 1442-1448. doi: 10.1038/sj.ijo.0803606

Question 3.10

Which of the following statements is not correct regarding the relation between obesity and renal disease?

a. Most common renal lesion seen in obese individuals is focal and segmental glomerulosclerosis and glomerulomegaly
b. Excessive weight gain may lead to decreased renal tubular sodium reabsorption and compensatory renal vasoconstriction
c. Proteinuria may develop in obese individuals due to nephron damage
d. High waist circumference has an association with poor renal function

The correct answer is "b."

All statements except "b." are correct. Weight gain leads to increased reabsorption of renal tubular sodium and compensatory renal vasodilatation.

Burton, J. O., Gray, L. J., Webb, D. R., Davies, M. J., Khunti, K., Crasto, W., . . . Brunskill, N. J. (2011). Association of anthropometric obesity measures with chronic kidney disease risk in a non-diabetic patient population. Nephrology Dialysis Transplantation, 27(5), 1860-1866. doi:10.1093/ndt/gfr574

Question 3.11

Which of the following statements is correct about the estimated glomerular filtration rate (GFR) in patients after bariatric surgery?

a. Estimated GFR remains one of the most reliable methods of renal function assessment
b. Estimated GFR does not depend on creatinine
c. Estimated GFR is likely to decrease in post-bariatric patients due to loss of muscle mass
d. Estimated GFR does not take into account the surface area of the patient
e. Estimated GFR may increase without real improvement of renal function

The correct answer is "e."

This interesting fact is derived from several observations. After bariatric surgery patients lose some muscle mass. Not only are GFR data tables obtained from patients who are not obese, the GFR calculations are not adjusted to decreased surface area after losing weight. This issue may lead to incorrect estimations of GFR. Some of the equations which are used in the assessment of GFR include CKD-EPI, MDRD, and Cockcroft-Gault. The later one incorporates lean body mass adjustments.

Editorial Board. (2016). Surgery for Obesity and Related Diseases, 12(1), I-Ii. doi:10.1016/s1550-7289(15)01029-1

Question 3.12

A 70-year-old patient undergoes gastric bypass surgery. His outcomes may differ from a 40-year-old who receives the same type of surgery. Which of the following statements is correct?

a. He is likely to have more excess weight loss
b. His chances to have complications are less
c. He has better chances to have remission of sleep apnea
d. Type 2 diabetes remission chances are higher
e. “a.” and “c.” are correct

The correct answer is "e."

Older age group has more chances of post-operative complications. Younger patients may see a remission of diabetes more often. However, older age group sees more excess weight loss and has better resolution of sleep apnea.

Question 3.13

A morbidly obese patient is investigated for sleep apnea as part of the preparative workup for bariatric surgery. A sleep study is ordered. His report shows six central apneas, 78 hypopneas, and an Apnea Hypopnea Index (AHI) of 17 per hour. Minimum oxygen saturation was 85%. In his follow-up visit with his family physician, the sleep study report was discussed. Which of the following statements is correct regarding his results?

a. His AHI index is normal
b. His AHI index indicates mild sleep apnea
c. His AHI index suggests moderate sleep apnea
d. His AHI index suggests severe sleep apnea
e. AHI is not particularly important in the prediction of sleep apnea

The correct answer is "c."

AHI less than 5 is normal and a value between 5 to 15 is considered mild. AHI between 15 to 30 is moderate and a value above 30 is regarded as severe. Recommendations in any such case are better sleep hygiene, weight loss, positional therapy, avoid alcohol and nicotine-containing products. Additionally, CPAP/BPAP titration is recommended to find the therapeutically effective positive pressure value. Sleep apnea could be central or obstructive.

In central apnea, cessation of the oral and nasal flow of air is observed simultaneously with cessation of respiratory movements for at least 10 seconds. On the other hand, in obstructive apnea the air flow stops in the presence of continuing respiratory movements.

Shamsuzzaman, Abu S. M., et al. “Obstructive Sleep Apnea.” Jama, vol. 290, no. 14, Aug. 2003, p. 1906., doi:10.1001/jama.290.14.1906.

Question 3.14

What is a true statement about the definition of hypopnea?

a. Decreased flow > 30% from baseline for 20 seconds

b. Decreased flow > 30% from baseline for 10 seconds

c. Decreased flow > 40% from baseline for 5 seconds

d. Decreased flow > 50% from baseline for 10 seconds

e. Decreased flow > 50% from baseline for 20 seconds

The correct answer is "b."

Decreased flow > 30% from the baseline for 10 seconds is considered significant to confirm the diagnosis of a hypopnea event.

Question 3.15

Morbid obesity has a close association with obstructive sleep apnea. Determining the Apnea-Hypopnea Index (AHI) is essential in assessing the magnitude of obstructive sleep apnea.
Which of the following statements is correct?

a. AHI = (numbers of apneas + numbers of hypopneas) / sleep hours

b. AHI = sleep hours / (numbers of apneas + numbers of hypopneas)

c. AHI = (numbers of apneas - numbers of hypopneas) / sleep hours

d. AHI = sleep hours / (numbers of apneas - numbers of hypopneas)

e. AHI= (numbers of apneas + numbers of hypopneas + Respiratory Effort Related Arousal (RERAs) / sleep hours

The correct answer is "a."

AHI is determined by the sum of the numbers of apneas and number of hypopneas, divided by sleep hours.

Question 3.16

Obstructive sleep apnea has a close association with morbid obesity. It can have many adverse effects. There is higher risk of developing several conditions if obstructive sleep apnea remains untreated. A morbidly obese patient with untreated sleep apnea can develop which of the following conditions?

a. Congestive heart failure (CHF)

b. Atrial fibrillation

c. Cerebrovascular events

d. Hypertension

e. Pulmonary hypertension

f. All above statements are correct

The correct answer is "f."

Obesity and sleep apnea have a close association. Endothelial damage via various mechanisms and repeated hypoxia leads to the production of oxidative stress. It can lead to enhanced atherosclerosis potential through the production of inflammatory cytokines.

Question 3.17

Several medications are known to affect lipid and carbohydrate metabolism. Which of the following medications may lead to hyperglycemia, lipid disorder, decreased subcutaneous fat, and more visceral fat accumulation?

a. Loop diuretics

b. Proton pump inhibitors

c. Antiretroviral therapy

d. Cephalosporins

e. Chronic coumadin use

The correct answer is "c."

Antiretroviral therapy is noted to have stated side effects. Metformin may help in preventing some of these effects.

Question 3.18

A 48-year-old female is considering bariatric surgery for her lifelong problem of morbid obesity. At this age, she is also struggling with her perimenopausal symptoms. She spends considerable time on the web in search for perimenopausal symptoms. At her next visit with her family physician, she asks several questions about osteoporosis at her age and the potential effect of weight loss surgery. The family physician discusses at length various aspects of osteoporosis. Please select the correct statement.

a. Weight loss with bariatric surgery will potentially cause her to lose bone mass density

b. Bone loss is more pronounced in perimenopausal women and older men

c. Trabecular bones lose more density as compared to other sites

d. Older individuals losing more than 10% of weight carry more risk of hip fracture

e. All the above statements are correct

The correct answer is "e."

Several studies have looked at the association of loss of bone density with weight loss. It potentially increases the risk of fractures in older individuals of both sexes. Hip and distal forearms are two common fracture sites in this group. Shapses, Sue A., and Deeptha Sukumar. Annual Review of Nutrition, U.S. National Library of Medicine, 21 Aug. 2012, www.ncbi.nlm.nih.gov/pmc/articles/PMC4016236/.

Question 3.19

A 39-year-old female with morbid obesity has abnormal liver functions for the last two years. She has a BMI of 53. Gastroenterology and bariatric consultations were requested. Liver biopsy was done. The histopathology report revealed 40% macrovesicular steatosis. A follow up visit was arranged with her physician and the severity of steatosis was explained to her. Please select the correct statement.

a. She has severe hepatic steatosis

b. She has moderate hepatic steatosis

c. She has mild hepatic steatosis

d. If ballooning degeneration is present, it is the characteristic sign of steatohepatitis

e. “b” and “d” statements are correct

The correct answer is "e."

On microscopic examination, less than 5% steatosis is considered normal. 5 to 33% is mild, 34 to 66% is moderate, and more than 66% is severe. Ballooning degeneration determines the presence of steatohepatitis.
“Nonalcoholic Steatohepatitis (NASH).” Pathology Outlines - PathologyOutlines.com,
www.pathologyoutlines.com/topic/liverNASH.html.

Psychology and Counseling Aspects

Question 4.1

Motivational interview (MI) is a crucial component of managing behavioral modification in patients suffering from obesity. Which of the following statements is not correct about the motivational interview?

a. It is a client-centered counseling style to elicit behavior change by clients to help explore and resolve ambivalence.

b. MI can result in more weight loss and better maintenance

c. Collaboration rather than confrontation is a key component of MI

d. Close-ended questions can easily discover the patient's participation, goals, and values

e. Clinician provides resources to the patients to bring change

f. Generating gap to highlight discrepancy in goal setting, and roll with resistance are essential aspects of the motivational interview.

The correct answer is "d."

Close-ended questions are not particularly useful in determining a patient's goals, values, and health beliefs. All other statements are true. Client-centered counseling, motivational interview, collaboration, provision of resources to patients to bring changes, and to generate gap to express discrepancy are effective strategies.

Roberts, R. E., Deleger, S., Strawbridge, W. J., & Kaplan, G. A. (2003). Prospective association between obesity and depression: evidence from the Alameda County Study. International Journal of Obesity, 27(4), 514-521. doi: 10.1038/sj.ijo.0802204

Question 4.2

Several different psychological approaches and therapies are available for patients seeking help with the problem of obesity. Which of the following statements is true?

a. Interpersonal therapy is an individualized approach with a focus to address emotional triggers and avoid relapsing into past habits

b. High prevalence of depression in obese patients requires screening on initial exam

c. Behavioral therapy has components involving positive and negative reinforcements

d. Cognitive therapy involves techniques to change ineffective thinking

e. Cognitive behavior therapy involves changes in cognitive understanding to enable the client to recognize various triggers which lead to self-defeating actions or behaviors

f. All the above statements are correct

The correct answer is "f."

Interpersonal, behavioral, cognitive, and cognitive behavior therapies are essential elements of psychological interventions. A high percentage of bariatric cases have depression. This issue needs to be assessed at the initial examination.

Perri, M. G. (2014). Effects of behavioral treatment on long-term weight loss: Lessons learned from the look AHEAD trial. Obesity, 22(1), 3-4. doi:10.1002/oby.20672

Question 4.3

Motivational interview (MI) involves several stages. Please select the statement stating correct order.

a. Action, preparation, contemplation, pre-contemplation, and relapse
b. Action, contemplation, preparation, pre-contemplation, and relapse
c. Contemplation, pre-contemplation, preparation, action, and relapse
d. Preparation, action, pre-contemplation, contemplation, and relapse

e. Pre-contemplation, contemplation, preparation, action, and relapse

The correct answer is "e."

Question 4.4

Motivational interview (MI) involves several components. A therapist uses a technique which can have variants including reflection, shifting focus, reframing, and siding with resistance. Please select the statement stating the type of technique described here.

a. Roll with resistance
b. Therapeutic paradox
c. Evocation
d. Collaboration
e. Pre-contemplation

The correct answer is "a."

Question 4.5

A 33-year-old female follows a bariatric practice. She weighs 325 lbs. She lives with her boyfriend and has several family stressors. She has six visits to the office in the last 14 months. At the start of the program, her weight was 324 lbs. She had a few appointments with the nutritionist too. Several medications to help her lose weight were tried at various times. The list of drugs includes phentermine, topiramate, and bupropion/naltrexone combination. She admits having several, poor eating habits. She likes cheese with crackers and consumes a large amount daily; it seems she is not willing to give up this habit. Her case was discussed in the multidisciplinary meeting of the practice and during her next visit, the counsellor tells her, "You have followed our program for a good amount of time. It looks as if you have too much going on in your life and it is not letting you make a change. I am wondering what our strategy could be going forward." Please select the statement which reflects the technique that the counsellor used on her to address the issue.

a. Roll with resistance

b. Therapeutic paradox

c. Evocation

d. Collaboration

e. Pre-contemplation

The correct answer is "b."

It is an example of a therapeutic paradox. The counselor comments and hopes that the patient may bring a thought or initiative to change the situation.

Question 4.6

A 37-year-old female joins a bariatric program. She is recently diagnosed with insulin resistance and impaired glucose tolerance. Her mother and one of the older sisters have diabetes. She is very scared of developing this disease. She makes a lot of dietary changes and goes to the gym regularly. She lost 20 labs in three months. At her follow up visit her doctor is pleased with her progress. He says "You have done very well. Can you tell what changes in diet and lifestyle helped you to lose this much of weight"?

Please select the technique reflected by his statement.

a. Roll with resistance

b. Therapeutic paradox

c. Affirmation

d. Collaboration

e. Pre-contemplation

The correct answer is "c."

It is an example of affirmation. These statements need to be real and relevant. Provider here recognizes the patient's strengths and effort to make a favorable change.

Investigations for an Obese Patient

Question 5.1

A morbidly obese patient is seen in the primary care physician's office. After history taking, a physical examination was done. The physician notices some skin changes with pigmentation and maculopapular lesions. Acanthosis nigricans is suspected. Which of the following statements is correct regarding this condition?

a. It is likely to be present on the face, the front of neck and chest.
b. HbA1c and glucose tolerance tests with fasting insulin levels should be done as part of the workup
c. The color of rash is likely red to blue
d. Rash is unlikely to be present on side or back of neck, axillae, or groins
e. None of the above statements are correct

The correct answer is "b."

The usual distribution of this dark and blackish pigmentation is at the back of neck, axillae, and groins. Prevalence of diabetes is high in this group of patients, thus blood glucose and HbA1c needs to be checked.

Hermanns-L T., Scheen, A., & Pierard, G. E. (2004). Acanthosis Nigricans Associated with Insulin Resistance. American Journal of Clinical Dermatology, 5(3), 199-203. doi:10.2165/00128071-200405030-00008

Question 5.2

On further examination, the physician notices that the patient has a large abdominal pannus. This pannus extends to cover the upper thighs. What grade will be assigned to this pannus while documenting it in findings?

a. Grade 1
b. Grade 2
c. Grade 3
d. Grade 4
e. Grade 5

The correct answer is "c."

A pannus extending to upper thighs is considered Grade 3. Other grades are as follows:

Grade 1 covers pubic hair; Grade 2 cover mons pubis; Grade 3 as stated above; Grade 4 extends to mid thighs; Grade 5 reaches the knees and beyond.

Panniculectomy Plastic Surgery Operation. (n.d.). Retrieved January 01, 2018, from http://www.bariatric-surgery.info/panniculectomy-surgical-procedure.htm

Question 5.3

The physician measures the blood pressure of the patient after selecting the appropriate size cuff. Which of the following statements is correct regarding blood pressure measurement of a morbidly obese patient?

a. The cuff should wrap less than one-third of the middle of the upper arm
b. The width of the cuff should not exceed arm diameter by 5%
c. The cuff should not wrap around two-thirds of the middle of the upper arm
d. Accurate reading cannot be taken with any blood pressure cuff
e. The width of the cuff should exceed diameter by 20%

The correct answer is "e."

The blood pressure readings may be falsely high if a smaller cuff is used for an obese patient. It is recommended that the bladder of the cuff should wrap around more than two-thirds of the middle of the upper arm and the width of the cuff should exceed 20 % of the diameter at the point of application. Upper arm circumference greater than 34 cm can be a used as an indication to select a larger cuff size. For pediatric patients, it is recommended that the patient should be sitting for at least 5 minutes before the reading is taken and their feet should be kept on the ground. The bladder of the cuff should cover more than 80% of the circumference of mid-arm. The width of the cuff should exceed mid-arm circumference by 40%.

Question 5.4

Regarding waist measurements, which of the following statements is correct?

a. The waist-hip circumference ratio of 0.7 in a male is a sign of central obesity
b. The waist is measured at the level of the iliac crest, while the patient is standing and at the end of expiration
c. The waist is measured while the patient is laying down with a deep breath in
d. The tape around the waist should be adequately snug around the skin with good compression
e. Waist to hip ratio of 1.2 defines it to be a gynecoid type of obesity with a strong association with metabolic syndrome

The correct answer is "b."

The point of measurement is just above hip bones, it should not be compressing the skin and should be placed horizontally. In American males, waist circumference of 40 inches (102 cm) or above and females 35 inches (88 cm) or above is considered as the cut-off for abdominal obesity. It should be noted that BMI correlates better with the metabolic disease as compared to waist circumference in patients with BMI ≥ 35kg/m^2. Cutoffs may be different for different racial and ethnic backgrounds.

Waist circumference of above 37 inches (94 cm) in middle aged males is a risk factor for development of type 2 diabetes and cardiovascular disease.

Assessing Your Weight. (2015, May 15). Retrieved December 28, 2017, from https://www.cdc.gov/healthyweight/assessing/Jacobson, Terry A., et al. "National Lipid Association Recommendations for Patient-Centered Management of Dyslipidemia: Part 1 – Executive Summary." Journal of Clinical Lipidology, vol. 8, no. 5, 2014, pp. 473–488., doi:10.1016/j.jacl.2014.07.007.

Question 5.5

Bioelectrical impedance (BIA) is commonly used in the workup of obese patients. Which of the following statements is correct regarding BIA?

a. It has an advantage ~~that~~ as it is not affected by the state of hydration

b. Fasting and recent exercise can alter BIA values

c. Fat mass has low impedance to flow of electric current

d. BIA has the advantage of being useful in extreme age groups

e. Low dose x-rays are used to measure the composition of body tissues

The correct answer is "b."

Bioelectrical impedance (BIA) is an estimate of body fat mass and fat-free mass. Fat of the body and other tissues differ in characteristics of electrical impedance. BIA is rapid, easy to use and have virtually no safety concerns. Fasting, old age, hydration status and exercise may affect the value of BIA.

Question 5.6

Which of the following statements is not correct about "Brown Adipose Tissue"?

a. Brown adipose tissue estimation can be done with PET scan
b. Lean individuals have more brown adipose content than obese individuals.
c. Three-fourths of brown adipose content is found in cervical, supraclavicular, and axillary areas
d. Brown adipose tissue may have a key role in energy expenditure
e. Obese individuals carry more brown adipose tissue

The correct answer is "e."

Steelman, G. M., & Westman, E. C. Evaluation of the obese patient. In: Steelman, G. M., & Westman, E. C. (Eds.) Obesity:

evaluation and treatment essentials, 2nd Edition. Boca Raton: CRC Press, Taylor & Francis Group Press; 2016, pp.77-79

Question 5.7

A 32-year-old woman was seen in her family doctor's office. A body fat analyzer was used to check her body composition. It was determined that she has 27% fat. Which of the following statements is correct?

a. She is likely to be an athlete
b. She should be regarded as obese
c. Her body fat percentage is not within an acceptable range
d. In women, 25 % of body fat is labeled as essential fat
e. If she loses 5% of her body fat, she would be in fitness range

The correct answer is "e."

American Council on exercise classification (based on expert opinion) states more than 32 % of body fat in women as obesity. Levels between 25 to 31 % are acceptable. Fitness requires a level between 21 to 24%. Athletes usually have 14 to 20 % of body weight as fat. For men, these figures are 6 to 13% for athletes, 14 to 17% for fitness, 18 to 24% as acceptable, and more than 25% is considered as obesity.

Author Natalie Digate Muth Health and Fitness Expert Natalie Digate Muth. "What Are the Guidelines for Percentage of

Body Fat Loss?" Body Fat Loss | Guidelines for Percentage of Body Fat Loss | ACE Blog, www.acefitness.org/education-and-resources/lifestyle/blog/112/what-are-the-guidelines-for-percentage-of-body-fat-loss.

Question 5.8

A 28-year-old man who is a professional football player is seen in his PCP's office. He does heavy exercise most of the days. His height is 5'11" and he carries a weight of 260 lbs. Please select the correct statement.

a. Waist circumference will be more reliable in accessing adiposity
b. BMI measurement would give an appropriate assessment about his body fat
c. Body fat percentage calculation will be a better measure to assess body composition
d. None of the above statements is true

The correct answer is "c."

In situations of very high muscle mass such as in bodybuilders or patients with sarcopenia, the body fat percentage determination is a more accurate method for assessing body composition.

Question 5.9

In the evaluation of a bariatric patient, several tools are used. Which of the following is not an evaluation tool for sleep apnea?

a. Berlin Questionnaire

b. Stop-Bang Questionnaire

c. Epworth Scale

d. PHQ-9 Screen

The correct answer is "d."

PHQ- 9 (Patient Health Questionnaire) is used to screen depression. Options "a., "b." and "c." are used to assess sleep apnea. Stop-Bang Scale looks at some of the symptoms like snoring, tiredness, observed sleep apnea, blood pressure, age, circumference of the neck, and gender.

Biological Plausibility Linking Sleep Apnea and Metabolic ... https://www.nature.com/articles/nrendo.2016.22

"PHQ-9 Depression Test Questionnaire." Patient.info, Patient.info, patient.info/doctor/patient-health-questionnaire-phq-9.

Question 5.10

Which of the following studies is not useful in the evaluation of body composition of a morbidly obese patient?

a. Dual-energy X-ray absorptiometry
b. Bioelectric impedance
c. Near-infrared interactance
d. QMR (quantitative magnetic resonance imaging)
e. Whole body air displacement plethysmography (BODPOD)
f. HIDA scan with CCK

The correct answer is "f."

HIDA scan with CCK is used to assess biliary and gallbladder function. All other items in statements “a.” to “e.” can be used to determine body fat composition.

Question 5.11

In evaluating an obese patient, it may be useful to have an assessment of fat-free mass and lean body mass. Please select the correct statement.

a. Lean body mass is total body mass minus fatty tissues. In a nonobese person it is generally 75% of total body mass

b. Fat-free mass is total body mass minus total body fat.

c. Lean body mass differs from the fat free mass by approximately 5%

d. Fat-free mass can be measured with techniques like dual-energy X-ray absorptiometry (DXA) scan or bioelectrical impedance (BIA)

e. All the above statements are correct

The correct answer is "e."

Fat-free mass is the sum of water, minerals, protein, and glycogen of body. On the other hand, lean body mass is the sum of water, mineral, protein, glycogen, fat in organs, bone marrow, and CNS.

Question 5.12

A 65-year-old lady who is status post gastric bypass 15 years ago. She lost about 90 lbs. after bariatric surgery. She did not prove to be a very compliant patient and has regained significant weight back over the course of years. She is evaluated with several tests and a few scans were ordered. One of her report states about T and Z scores. She looked her reports at the online portal for her records. At the follow-up visit, she has questions about these scores. Please select the correct statement.

a. T and Z scores determine cardiovascular risk.
b. T and Z scores determine diabetes development risk
c. T and Z scores determine depression development risk
d. T and Z scores determine osteoporosis development risk
e. T and Z scores determine renal failure development risk

The correct answer is "d."

T and Z scores determine risk for osteoporosis. DXA scans can be used to identify this risk. Patients who are post-bariatric surgery, especially those who have gastric bypass, have a significant risk of osteoporosis. A T-score in range of -1 to -2.5 is regarded as osteopenia, and a score of -2.5 or below reflects osteoporosis. Normal level is -1 and above.

T-score compares the bone density of an individual with a 30-year-old healthy person of the same gender whereas Z score compares bone density with an average person of same gender and age.

Question 5.13

Measurements of basal and resting energy expenditure may provide useful insights into the management of obese patients. Please select the correct statement regarding calorimetry.

a. Indirect calorimetry is done while the patient is in a chamber and measures the difference of the temperature of water entering and exiting the chamber

b. Direct calorimetry estimates the energy expenditure by estimating consumption and production of oxygen and carbon dioxide respectively

c. Respiratory quotient (RQ) = O_2consumed/CO_2 produced

d. An RQ of 1.4 means lipolysis with underfeeding

e. RQ of fats is 0.7

The correct answer is "e."

Indirect calorimetry is done with measurements of carbon dioxide produced and oxygen consumed. RQ for carbs and fats is 1 and 0.7, respectively. Low RQ is seen in ketosis. Its value is high in conditions of overfeeding and lipogenesis. RQ value below 0.85 reflects underfeeding. Respiratory Quotient (RQ) = CO_2 produced/O_2 consumed.

Sabounchi, N S, et al. "Best-Fitting Prediction Equations for Basal Metabolic Rate: Informing Obesity Interventions in Diverse Populations." International Journal of Obesity, vol. 37, no. 10, 2013, pp. 1364–1370., doi:10.1038/ijo.2012.218.

Question 5.14

Morbid obesity adversely affects the dynamics of breathing. Please select the correct statement.

a. Respiratory compliance is increased
b. Work of breathing is decreased
c. Functional residual capacity is increased
d. Closing volume to functional vital capacity ratio is high
e. Closing volume to functional vital capacity ratio is low

Correct answer is "e. "

In morbid obesity the respiratory compliance is decreased. The primary contributing factor is chest wall compliance. Recumbent position also adversely affects the condition. Work of breathing is increased with a decrease of functional residual capacity. Low ratio for closing volume explains the predisposition to atelectasis. This becomes clinically relevant in post-operative settings.

Question 5.15

Morbid obesity alters several respiratory dynamics and pulmonary function values. Please select the correct statement.

a. FEV1 is likely to be high in an obese individual
b. FEV1 is likely to be low in an obese patient
c. FEV1 is likely to be the same for normal and morbidly obese individuals.
d. In obese individuals, relationship between respiratory resistance and functional residual capacity (FRC) is linear

Correct answer is "b."

FEV1 is likely to be low in obese individuals and an inverse relationship exists between respiratory resistance and FRC.

Krishnan Parameswaran, MD PhD FRCP FCCP, David C Todd, MD FRCPC, and Mark Soth, MD FRCPC
Author information Copyright and License information Disclaimer
This article has been cited by other articles in PMC.

Question 5.16

A super morbidly obese patient is seen in the pulmonary office. He has a BMI of 72. He is suspected to have obesity hypoventilation syndrome (OHS). The pulmonologist is interested in checking his respiratory muscle endurance. Which pulmonary function value can correlate objectively with respiratory muscle endurance measurements?

a. Maximal voluntary ventilation (MVV)
b. FEV1
c. FRC
d. Baseline VO_2
e. Respiratory rate

Correct answer is "a."

MVV can be used as a measure of respiratory muscle endurance. In otherwise healthy obese patients, it may be reduced by 20%. A reduction by 45% may be observed in patients with OHS. Several mechanisms are proposed in this instance. Overstretching of muscle fibers, spine position, and diaphragmatic dysfunction related to increased abdominal fat could be responsible for this effect.

Sharp JT, Druz WS, Kondragunta VR. Diaphragmatic response to body position changes in obese patients with obstructive sleep apnea. Am Rev Respir Dis. 1986;133:32–7.

Question 5.17

Obese patients generally show poor performance related to high breathing effort tasks when doing pulmonary function tests (PFTs). MVV is a test requiring high breathing efforts. Please select the correct statement regarding expected findings in a morbidly obese patient while performing MVV.

a. Slow and deep breathing pattern is observed
b. Relative dead space (VD)/Tidal volume (VT) ratio is increased
c. Relative dead space (VD)/Tidal volume (VT) ratio is decreased
d. Rapid breathing is more economical in terms of O_2 consumption

Correct answer is "b."

In normal subjects, oxygen consumption (VO_2) attributed to respiratory work is less than 3% of the total body consumption of O_2 during quiet breathing. In obese patients, the cost of O_2 may increase to four folds and O_2 consumption increases by 70%. Relative dead space increases and tidal volume tends to fall making the ratio higher.

Koenig SM. Pulmonary complications of obesity. Am J Med Sci. 2001;321:249–79.

Question 5.18

Select the correct statement about effects of obesity on lung volumes.

a. Expiratory reserve volume (ERV) is increased
b. Expiratory reserve volume (ERV) is decreased
c. Residual volume (RV) is decreased
d. RV to total lung capacity (TLC) ratio is decreased
e. Expiratory reserve volume is increased in supine position

Correct answer is “b.”

ERV is likely to be decreased in a morbidly obese patient. This reduction is most observed in supine position. Vital capacity (VC) and total lung capacity (TLC) are usually within normal range in an average obese patient. Residual volume (RV), RV to TLC ratio, resting expenditure of energy, and minute ventilation values are increased. Spirometry shows obstructive effect in severely obese patients. Restrictive effect is seen in mild to moderate forms of obesity.

Ray CS, Sue DY, Bray G, Hansen JE, Wasserman K. Effects of obesity on respiratory function. Am Rev Respir Dis. 1983;128:501–6.

Inselma LS, Milanese A, Deurloo A. Effect of obesity on pulmonary function in children. Pediatr Pulmonol. 1993;16:130–7.

Question 5.19

Carbon monoxide diffusion capacity (DLCO) has a relationship with weight in obese patients. Similarly, a relationship exists between DLCO and alveolar volume. Please select the correct statement regarding this relationship.

a. Weight loss increases DLCO and DLCO to alveolar volume ratio
b. Weight gain decreases DLCO and DLCO to alveolar volume ratio
c. Weight gain increases DLCO and DLCO to alveolar volume ratio
d. DLCO is inversely related to lung volume measurement
e. A high DLCO and DLCO ratio is seen in in atelectasis

Correct answer is "c."

DLCO value relates directly to lung volume measurement. High DLCO values are seen in otherwise healthy obese patients. Low DLCO and DLCO to alveolar volume ratio is seen in conditions with loss of pulmonary capillary bed, such as atelectasis.

Ray CS, Sue DY, Bray G, Hansen JE, Wasserman K. Effects of obesity on respiratory function. Am Rev Respir Dis. 1983;128:501–6.

Question 5.20

In healthy subjects, ventilation and perfusion has a specific pattern of distribution. Please select the correct statement.

a. In normal weight subjects, ventilation is lowest in dependent zones
b. In obese patients, ventilation may be highest in nondependent zones and there is more perfusion in dependent zones.
c. In obese patients, perfusion may be predominantly to upper lung zones.
d. Expiratory reserve volume (ERV) bears no relationship to ventilation perfusion ratio in obese patients

Correct answer is "b."

In otherwise normal subjects, ventilation is highest in dependent lung zones. ERV can be decreased in obese subjects resulting in ventilation shifting to upper zones. Airway closure with alveolar collapse could be the reason for underventilation of lung bases.

Holley HS, Milic-Emili J, Becklake MR, Bates DV. Regional distribution of pulmonary ventilation and perfusion in obesity. J Clin Invest. 1967;46:475–81

Question 5.21

The graphs (Figure 2) reflect information about one of the lung volumes in a normal person and in different clinical situations, including a morbidly obese subject who is otherwise healthy. This lung volume is plotted against time. Looking at the graph, which of the lung volumes is likely shown?

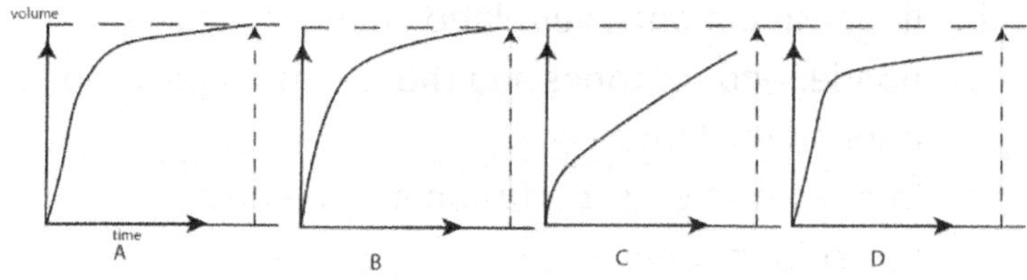

Figure 2

a. Residual volume
b. Forced vital capacity (FVC)
c. Inspiratory reserve volume
d. Tidal volume

Correct answer is "b."

Question 5.22

Pertaining to the question above, which of the graphs (Figure 2) will be typically seen in a morbidly obese patient who is otherwise healthy.

a. Curve A
b. Curve B
c. Curve C
d. Curve D

Correct answer is "d."

Question 5.23

The patient in the question above is planning to undergo bariatric surgery. His current BMI is 58. Select correct statement.

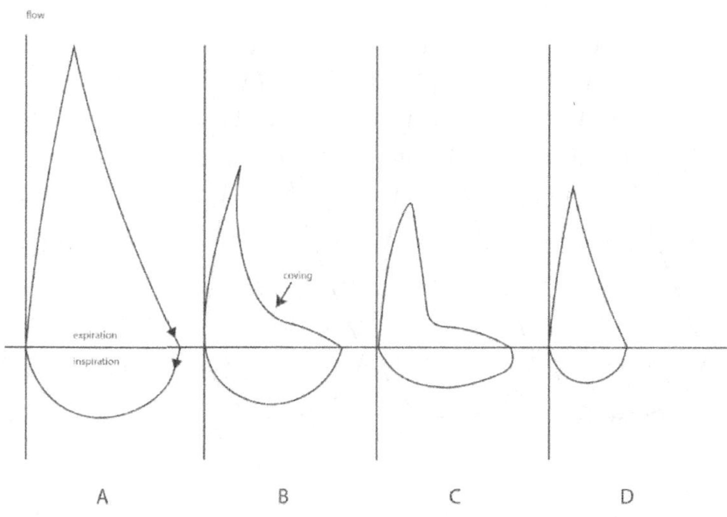

Figure 3

a. His curve of spirometry will more likely be like D
b. His curve of spirometry will more likely be like C
c. Coving seen in the curve is a specific phenomenon seen in morbidly obese patients
d. He is likely to have smaller area under the curve after losing substantial weight

Correct answer is “a.”

Question 5.24

Select the curve (figure 3) which will likely be seen in a morbidly obese patient who loses 95% of excess weight with no history of smoking or bronchial asthma

a. Curve A
b. Curve B
c. Curve C
d. Curve D

Correct answer is “a.”

Graph A is for a normal subject. Graph B shows relationship in a person with mild COPD with obstructive pattern. Once obstructive lung disease gets worse, appearance of graph becomes as shown in C. Coving effect is seen in obstructive airway disease. Morbid obesity leads to predominantly restrictive effects. Shape of the loop remains preserved (Graph D). Coving is typically seen in severe COPD cases. Area under the curve is likely to increase after weight loss following bariatric surgery.

Question 5.25

Which of the volumes is affected most in morbid obesity?

a. Td (Tidal volume)
b. TLC (Total lung volume)
c. ERV (Expiratory reserve volume)
d. RV (Residual volume)

Correct answer is “c.”
In obese patients, a decrease in Expiratory Reserve Volume is the most seen abnormality. This is thought to be due to decreased functional residual capacity due to the mass loading effect of obesity. TLC and RV are not expected to change much in this situation. Supine position pushes the diaphragm up, leading to fall in ERV.

Ray CS, Sue DY, Bray G, Hansen JE, Wasserman K. Effects of obesity on respiratory function. Am Rev Respir Dis.

Question 5.26

Fat distribution in the body influences pulmonary function. Which of the following is more closely related to adverse effect on pulmonary function?

a. Abdominal obesity
b. Obesity of lower extremities
c. Back
d. In older people the relationship between distribution of fat pattern and pulmonary function is stronger

Correct answer is “a.”

Abdominal obesity is more closely related to pulmonary function abnormality in obese subjects. This effect diminishes with advancing age. It is suggested that abdominal circumference to hip breadth ratio and subscapular skin fold thickness can be objectively related to FEV1 and FVC abnormalities.

Lazarus R, Sparrow D, Weiss ST. Effects of obesity and fat distribution on ventilatory function. Chest. 1997;111:891–8.

Question 5.27

Pulmonary function test report of an obese patient before bariatric surgery reveals forced vital capacity of 2.52 liter (It is 76% of predicted). FEV-1 is 2.09 liters. (78% of predicted) FEV-1/FVC ratio is normal at 83%. FEV (25-75%) is 73% of the predicted value. Slow vital capacity is 2.12 liters (64 % of predicted). Select the correct statement.

a. Report shows mild sleep apnea.
b. Mild obstructive ventilatory defect is present
c. Restrictive disease cannot be ruled out
d. None of the above statements is correct
e. Statements b and c are correct

Correct answer is (e)

The data shown in the question reflects mild obstructive ventilatory defect. The data does not rule out restrictive disease.

Question 5.28

Resting energy expenditure (REE) estimation has a role in understanding and management of obesity. Please select the correct statement about REE / Basal metabolic rate (BMR)

a. Harris-Benedict equation can be used to assess BMR
b. Schofield formula is most accurate in assessing BMR
c. Cunningham's formula gives the best BMR estimations
d. Indirect calorimetry is the most widely available and used method

Correct answer is "a."

Various formulas including Harris – Benedict equation can be used for the determination of resting energy expenditure. Its accuracy may vary for different BMI ranges. Equipment used to implement indirect calorimetry is expensive and not widely available.

Lee, Sun Hee, and Eun Kyung Kim. "Accuracy of predictive equations for resting metabolic rates and daily energy expenditures of police officials doing shift work by type of work." *Clinical nutrition research* vol. 1,1 (2012): 66-77. doi:10.7762/cnr.2012.1.1.66

Question 5.29

A morbidly obese patient is seen by pulmonologist. Spirometry was done. The report states that forced vital capacity (FVC), FEV1, and FEV1/FVC are normal. There is no significant response to bronchodilator administration. The diffusion capacity is moderately reduced. Expiratory reserve volume (ERV) is reduced and DLCO overcorrects with alveolar volume. The TLC is moderately reduced. Select the correct statement.

a. It suggests predominantly obstructive disease
b. It suggests predominantly restrictive disease
c. It suggests neither obstructive nor restrictive disease
d. The facts given are insufficient to comment on obstructive or restrictive disease pattern.

Correct answer is "b."

Restrictive lung disease is commonly seen in morbidly obese patients who are otherwise normal.

Question 5.30

A patient with BMI of 53 is found to have abnormal liver functions. On abdominal ultrasound fatty infiltration of the liver was suspected. A percutaneous core needle liver biopsy was done by the interventional radiologist.
The biopsy demonstrates steatosis score of 2 out of 3. lobular inflammatory score of 3 out of 3 and balloon cells (score 1 of 2). Total score 6 out of 8. A Trichrome stain revealed hepatic cirrhosis (fibrosis stage 4 of 4). An Iron stain was negative. A Reticulin stain demonstrates preservation of the reticulin framework. Based on the report stated, select the correct statement.

a. Patient has steatohepatitis with cirrhosis
b. Balloon cells confirm liver cell injury
c. Lobular inflammation confirms steatohepatitis
d. A score of 0-2 means no nonalcoholic steatohepatitis (NASH).
e. A score of above 5 is definite NASH
f. All above statements are correct.

Correct answer is "f."

Steatosis of less than 5% is scored 0 and more than 66% is scored as 3. Similarly, for ballooning a score of 0 is assigned for no ballooning and 2 is for citing many ballooning cells. For lobular inflammation, a score of 0 to 3 is used. More than 4 foci of inflammation per field is scored as 3. NAFLD activity score (NAS) is determined by combining all the three category scores.
https://www.nature.com/articles/3800680/tables/3 Retrieved on 12/8/2019

Question 5.31

Abdominal ultrasound is requested for a patient with BMI of 57. He has abnormal liver enzymes. AST and ALT were moderately elevated. Fatty liver disease is suspected. Which of the following sonographic findings will be suggestive of fatty liver disease?

a. Decreased brightness at the surface of liver
b. Increased brightness at 4 to 5 cm deep in liver
c. Hyperechoic 4 to 5 cm deep in liver
d. Hypoechoic at the surface of liver

Correct answer is "b."

Diagnostic accuracy of NAFLD increases if at least 4 out of 5 sonographic features are present. These include attenuation of image quickly within 4-5 cm of depth, diffuse echogenicity with brightness within the first 2-3 cm of depth, liver being uniformly heterogeneous, thick subcutaneous depth {> 2 cm}, and no visible edges of liver with entire field filled with liver

Riley TR, Mendoza A, Bruno MA. Bedside ultrasound can predict nonalcoholic fatty liver disease in the hands of clinicians using a prototype image. Dig Dis Sci. 2006;51:982–985.

Question 5.32

Ultrasound of liver is requested for a patient seeking bariatric surgery. Sonographer report shows hyperechoic liver. What could be the interpretation with this echo pattern?

a. Her liver is normal
b. Liver has fatty infiltration
c. Liver is grossly cirrhotic
d. Ultrasound accuracy of picking up fatty liver disease is best when less than 5 % of liver parenchyma is involved with fatty change.

Correct answer is "b."

Hyperechoic image of ultrasound suggests fatty infiltration of liver. Advanced cirrhotic liver may show hypoechoic nodules. Normal liver may contain up to 5% of fat in the parenchyma. Ultrasound is reported to have sensitivity of 84.8% and specificity of 93.6% for diagnosing fatty liver if steatosis is ≥ 20 to 30%.

Hernaez, Ruben et al. "Diagnostic accuracy and reliability of ultrasonography for the detection of fatty liver: a meta-analysis." *Hepatology (Baltimore, Md.)* vol. 54,3 (2011): 1082-1090. doi:10.1002/hep.24452

Question 5.33

Fiberoscan is a test utilized in clinical settings. Select the correct statement.

a. A test to check clot strength
b. A test to check muscle fiber strength
c. A test to check fatty liver
d. A test to check joint ligaments

Correct answer is “c.”

Fibroscan is a relatively newer technique to assess liver disease. It uses 50-MHz ultrasound wave. As the wave passes through liver parenchyma, measurement of shear wave velocity gives estimation of liver stiffness in kilopascals (kPa). Liver stiffness corelates fairly with liver fibrosis or cirrhosis. Regular ultrasound has a sensitivity of 71% to detect liver cirrhosis whereas fibroscan can detect it in almost 100% of cases. In normal subjects, stiffness measures 2.6 to 6.1 kPa for males and 2.3 to 5.8 kPa for females. A score of 7.2 kPa or above is suggestive of significant fibrosis. Cirrhosis may show a score over 14.5 kPa.

Question 5.34

Ultrasound examination of liver was done for a morbidly obese patient. A specific comment about liver echogenicity was made. Select the correct statement.

a. Echogenicity is likely to be high
b. Echogenicity is likely to be low
c. In fatty liver echogenicity is not altered
d. Routine ultrasound is the best test to comment on liver fibrosis

Correct answer is "a."

Fatty livers show more echogenicity on sonogram. Fibroscan is a newer high frequency device used in assessing liver stiffness by estimating propagation velocity of a shear wave through liver parenchyma. It can predict liver fibrosis more accurately.

Pathik, Parikh et al. "Fibroscan versus simple noninvasive screening tools in predicting fibrosis in high-risk nonalcoholic fatty liver disease patients from Western India." *Annals of gastroenterology* vol. 28,2 (2015): 281-286.

Question 5.35

Morbid obesity and fatty liver disease share a close link. Liver biopsy remains an important evaluation tool in workup of fatty liver disease. Methodology of biopsy can affect pathology results. Please select the correct statement/s.

a. 2 cm or more of the core with at least 11 complete portal tracks are generally considered adequate specimen by most pathologists
b. Wedge biopsy is superior to a core biopsy
c. Wedge biopsies may under-represent fibrosis
d. Prolonged anesthesia time can produce "surgical hepatitis" because of anesthetic gases
e. Options "a" and "d" are correct

Correct answer is "e."

Amount of liver specimen collected, and its location can affect the results. Adequate core biopsy seems to provide enough representative tissue for better interpretation of histopathology. Prolonged anesthesia may cause infiltrates of leukocytes resulting in "surgical hepatitis".

Ratziu V, Charlotte F, Heurtier A, *et al*. Sampling variability of liver biopsy in nonalcoholic fatty liver disease. *Gastroenterology* 2005;**128**:1898–1906.

Question 5.36

Variability exists among the pathologists for the diagnostic interpretation of liver biopsy specimens for fatty liver. There are some criteria which are agreed by most experts. Fat alone or fat and inflammation with evidence of ballooning are the most accepted criteria. Please select the correct statement

a. Fat with inflammation confirms the diagnosis of NAFLD (Nonalcoholic fatty liver disease)
b. Fat with inflammation confirms the diagnosis of NASH (Nonalcoholic steatohepatitis)
c. Fat with inflammation and ballooning confirms the diagnosis of NAFLD
d. Presence of fibrosis in zone 3 (perisinusoidal) points to NAFLD but not NASH

Correct answer is "a."

Presence of ballooning of cells qualifies for the diagnosis of NASH. Presence of fibrosis in zone 3 of sinusoids is indicative of past or active NASH.

Question 5.37

Morbid obesity has a close link with fatty liver disease. Differentiation by liver biopsy between nonalcoholic fatty liver disease (NAFLD) and alcoholic steatohepatitis (ASH) can be difficult in some cases. There are few differences which can be appreciated on histology. Please select the correct statement.

a. Mallory hyalines are common in nonalcoholic steatohepatitis (NASH)
b. Mallory hyalines are common in alcoholic steatohepatitis (ASH)
c. Neutrophilic infiltrates are more common in NASH
d. Foamy degeneration is common in NSAH

Correct answer is "b."

Mallory hyaline and neutrophilic infiltrates are common histological findings in ASH.

Question 5.38

Insulin resistance is associated with several distinct effects and associations. It is linked with weight gain and morbid obesity. Please select the correct statement about insulin resistance.

a. Decreased level of C-reactive protein is observed when insulin level is raised
b. Increased levels of adiponectin are seen in insulin resistance

c. low-density lipoprotein (LDL) particle size tends to become larger
d. Decreased atherogenic risk
e. Intermittent fasting may help reduce insulin resistance

Correct answer is "e."

Increased level of C-reactive protein, decreased adiponectin, reduced size of low -density lipoprotein particles and increased atherogenic risk is seen with insulin resistance. Beneficial role of intermittent fasting is observed in insulin resistance.

Question 5.39

Which of the following statements about fatty liver is true?

a. Patients with type 1 diabetes have higher risk of developing fatty liver than patients with type 2 diabetes
b. Insulin resistance is not a risk factor for developing fatty liver
c. NASH decreases the risk of hepatocellular carcinoma
d. ALT level of above 19 in women and more than 30 in men has a high association with fatty liver

Correct answer is “d.”

Patients with type 2 diabetes have higher risk of developing fatty liver disease. Risk for developing hepatocellular carcinoma is higher with NASH. Insulin resistance is also recognized as a risk factor. High ALT level is correlated with elevated risk of fatty liver.

Principles of Dietary Management

Question 6.1

A morbidly obese patient is suggested to go on a low-carb and low-calorie diet

Which of the following statements is correct?

a. A reduction of fasting insulin level is expected
b. Insulin / Glucagon ratio is likely to increase
c. The glycolytic/ lipogenic ratio is increased
d. Nutritional ketosis is anticipated if dietary intake is 150 to 200 grams of carbohydrates
e. In ketosis, dominant fuel for energy is amino acids

The correct answer is "a."

Reduction in insulin level is observed once patients are started on low-carb and low-calorie diets. Nutritional ketosis is seen when 50 gm or less of carbohydrates are ingested per day. Even three to five percent of sustained weight loss is proven to produce significant health benefits, and risks of developing diabetes may reduce by 30% or more.

Phinney, S., Bistrian, B., Wolfe, R., & Blackburn, G. (1983). The human metabolic response to chronic ketosis without caloric restriction: Physical and biochemical adaptation. Metabolism, 32(8), 757-768. doi:10.1016/0026-0495(83)90105-1

Question 6.2

Patients on low-carb diets develop state of ketosis. Which of the following statements is correct?

a. Blood pH is likely to be low with significant metabolic acidosis

b. Cardiac and skeletal muscles cannot use ß hydroxybutyric acid and acetoacetic acid as a source of energy

c. Decreased activity of hormone-sensitive lipase is expected

d. Urine output is likely to fall

e. Dietary adherence can be checked with breath acetone monitoring

f. All the above statements are correct

The correct answer is "e."

Orthostatic symptoms can appear due to diuresis related to ketone bodies and other mechanisms. The patient may be required to adjust their sodium intake and antihypertensive medications. Similarly, monitoring for gout and blood sugar is needed. Pancreatitis risk is increased if patients with chylomicronemia take low carb and high-fat diets.

Buse, G. J., Riley, K. D., Dress, C. M., & Neumaster, T. D. (2004). Patient with gemfibrozil-controlled hypertriglyceridemia that developed acute pancreatitis after starting ketogenic diet. Current Surgery, 61(2), 224-226. doi:10.1016/s0149-7944(03)00159-4

Question 6.3

A morbidly obese patient with 45 BMI is placed on a low-carb diet for weight loss. He has hypertension and obstructive sleep apnea. He does not have diabetes. His physician ordered urine analysis which shows ketones. Which of the following statements is correct?

a. It is imperative to limit sodium in the diet
b. His renal sodium excretion will be increased
c. Nutritional ketosis and starvation are similar regarding the loss of lean muscle mass
d. Urine output is likely to decrease
e. A decreased diuresis is expected in nutritional ketosis

The correct answer is "b."

Renal sodium excretion in ketosis is increased due to decreased serum insulin levels and osmotic effects or urinary ketone bodies.

Question 6.4

Low carbohydrate diet produces which of the following effects?

a. High-density lipoprotein (HDL) levels may rise
b. Increased triglycerides.
c. Significant reduction in low-density lipoproteins (LDL)
d. A considerable decrease in cholesterol
e. Weight Watchers, Jenny Craig and Nutrisystem, are typical examples of low carbohydrate diets

The correct answer is "a."

HDL is expected to be increased with low carbohydrate diets. Triglycerides are likely to be reduced. LDL and cholesterol are not affected significantly. The diets like South Beach and Aitkin are typically considered low carbohydrate diets. Weight Watchers, Jenny Craig and Nutrisystem, are low-calorie diets.

Question 6.5

Low-calorie diets are used as an option for weight loss. Which of the following statements is true regarding low-calorie diets?

a. Nutritional ketosis is observed

b. Cardiac and metabolic risks are reduced

c. Lean muscle mass is likely to be preserved.

d. Examples of low-calorie diets include South Beach and Atkins

e. Low calorie and low carb diets do not have similar cardiovascular risk reductions

The correct answer is "e."

The low-calorie diets do not produce nutritional ketosis. Their cardiovascular benefits are less pronounced as well.

Question 6.6

Which of the following statements is true about very low-calorie diets (VLCD)?

a. Daily calories are restricted to 1200 to 1600
b. Very low-calorie diets are available as only prepared formulas
c. The initial weight loss, especially in the first week, is mainly through loss of body fat
d. VLCDs are very palatable
e. The natriuresis seen with VLCD is due to insulin reduction and mobilization of liver and muscle glycogen

The correct answer is "e."

The initial loss of weight is due to diuresis, insulin reduction and moving water with glycogen breakdown. Daily calories are restricted to less than 800 kcal. These diets should be used in the supervision of trained clinicians.

Tsai, A. G., & Wadden, T. A. (2006). The Evolution of Very-Low-Calorie Diets: An Update and Meta-analysis*. Obesity, 14(8), 1283-1293. doi:10.1038/oby.2006.146

Question 6.7

A morbidly obese patient is enrolled in a medically supervised diet program. A low-calorie and high protein dietary plan was given. Which of the following statements is correct?

a. Orthostatic symptoms observed may be due to sodium deficiency requiring replacement of sodium

b. Gout may precipitate due to a renal mechanism involving competition of uric acid and beta-hydroxybutyric acid in renal tubules

c. Diabetic patients need attention and require adjustments in insulin doses with glucose monitoring

d. Hypertriglyceridemia of chylomicron origin is a contraindication for low-carbohydrate and high-fat diets

e. All the above statements are correct

The correct answer is "e."

All the above statements are correct. Orthostatic symptoms can appear due to diuresis, and this is seen because of ketone bodies and other mechanisms. Patients may need to adjust sodium intake and antihypertensive medications. Moreover, monitoring for gout and blood sugar is needed. Pancreatitis risk increases if patients with chylomicronemia take low carb and high-fat diets.

Buse, G. J., Riley, K. D., Dress, C. M., & Neumaster, T. D. (2004). Patient with gemfibrozil-controlled hypertriglyceridemia that developed acute pancreatitis after starting ketogenic diet. Current Surgery, 61(2), 224-226. doi:10.1016/s0149-7944(03)00159-4

Question 6.8

USDA Dietary reference intake (DRI) references protein intake as

a. 0.1 to 0.5 gm/kg/day
b. 0.8 to 2.0 gm/kg/day
c. 3 to 5 gm/kg/day
d. 6 to 8 gm/kg/day
e. 9 to 10 gm/kg/day

The correct answer is "b."

Protein requirement is 0.8 to 2.0 gm/kg/day. For fats DRI (USDA) is 30 gm/day

"Read 'Dietary Reference Intakes for Energy, Carbohydrate, Fiber, Fat, Fatty Acids, Cholesterol, Protein, and Amino Acids' at NAP.edu." National Academies Press: OpenBook, www.nap.edu/read/10490/chapter/12.

Question 6.9

A 45-year-old male with BMI 32 is seen in his family doctor's office. After annual physical and review of his lab panel, it is determined that he has abnormal lipids. His LDL is raised as is cholesterol. HDL is low. Triglycerides are elevated two folds the normal value. Appropriate advice is given to him. Please select the correct statement.

a. Reduced dietary intake of fats may lead to an increase in LDL
b. Dietary restriction of carbohydrates may lead to a greater decrease in triglycerides
c. Reduced dietary intake of fats may lead to a greater decrease of triglycerides
d. Dietary restriction of carbohydrates may lead to a greater reduction of LDLs.
e. A1c and sugar numbers are more related to fat intake rather than carbohydrate intake

The correct answer is "b."

Triglycerides numbers decrease more once carbohydrates are reduced in the diet. HDL numbers tend to increase. On the other hand, low-fat diets lead to decrease LDL and cholesterol levels. A1c and sugar values are more linked to carbohydrates.

Question 6.10

A morbidly obese patient is started on a very low carbohydrate diet. Please select the correct choice.

a. Typically, very low carbohydrate means less than 50 grams of carbohydrates
b. Very low carb diets generally contain 100 to 150 grams of carbohydrates
c. Very low carb containing diets have 160 to 200 grams of carbohydrates.
d. Very low carb containing diets do not need close supervision of the patient
e. Blood pressure is likely to increase in patients on very low carbohydrate containing diets.

The correct answer is "a."

Very low-carbohydrate diets contain less than 50 grams of carbohydrates typically. On the other hand, low-fat diets achieve 10 to 30% of calories from fats. Very low-calorie diets target at below 800 kcal/day. These kinds of diets require medical supervision.

Question 6.11

A morbidly obese patient is placed on a diet plan which allows her to take up to 20 grams of carbohydrates at the start of the program. It allows her to take fish, chicken, and beef. The patient is restricted from using processed foods with high glycemic index and foods containing trans fats. Which of the following diet plan is likely selected in this case?

a. Weight watchers
b. Mediterranean diet
c. TLC (therapeutic lifestyle change diet)
d. Atkins diet
e. Ornish diet

The correct answer is "d."

This diet profile points to Atkin diet plan. It includes several phases of implementation. It starts from induction and ends with a maintenance phase. Twenty grams of carbs are allowed in induction with encouragement to take more meats like beef, chicken, and fish. In the maintenance phase, 60 to 90 grams of carbs are allowed.
Mediterranean diet has more of natural components like grains, fruits, vegetables, and pulses. It emphasizes on the reduced intake of processed /high-fat diets and red meats. Medlife index can be a useful tool to check for compliance with the diet program. It includes physical activity and social interactions in the scoring system. Another method to check adherence to diet program is (MEDAS – Mediterranean Diet Adherence Screener).

"How Does a Low Carb Diet Work." Atkins, www.atkins.com/how-it-works.

Question 6.12

A morbidly obese patient with BMI of 57 undergoes Roux-en-Y gastric bypass for morbid obesity. He was readmitted with a leak from gastrojejunostomy anastomosis. He was taken to operating room, and abdominal washout was performed. A feeding tube was placed in the excluded stomach. The patient is subsequently managed in the surgical intensive care unit with ventilatory support. A nutritional consultation was requested. In the determination of his caloric goals, a discussion was made with the dietitian. Please select the correct statement regarding the caloric needs.

a. 22 to 25 kcal/kg of adjusted body weight
b. 11 to 14 kcal/kg of actual body weight
c. 22 to 25 kcal /kg of actual body weight
d. 22 to 25 kcal/kg of ideal body weight
e. 11 to 14 kcal/kg of ideal body weight
f. BMI can be used as the best index to calculate calories in this case

The correct answer is "d."

Option "d." is correct regarding the requirements of calories in this case. Societies of critical care and parenteral/enteral nutrition have laid guidelines for morbidly obese patients in ICU settings. Use of BMI and adjusted weights are not favored by these society recommendations. Indirect calorimeter measurements may be helpful. The recommendations include 11 to 14 kcal/kg of actual weight-based estimation if BMI is between 30 to 40. For BMI more than 50, ideal weight should be used to calculate the nutritional requirements.

"Intensive Care Enteral Nutrition in 2017." Relias Media - Continuing Medical Education Publishing, www.reliasmedia.com/articles/141452-intensive-care-enteral-nutrition-in-2017.

McClave, S A, et al. "Guidelines for the Provision and Assessment of Nutrition Support Therapy in the Adult Critically Ill Patient: Society of Critical Care Medicine (SCCM) and American Society for Parenteral and Enteral Nutrition (A.S.P.E.N.)." JPEN. Journal of Parenteral and Enteral Nutrition., U.S. National Library of Medicine, www.ncbi.nlm.nih.gov/pubmed/19398613.

Role of Physical Activity in Management of Obesity

Question 7.1

Which of the following statements is true regarding the need of physical activity in weight maintenance?

a. People doing 150 to 250 minutes of moderate intensity physical activity per week are likely to have a stable weight profile

b. A steady weight is regarded as up to 10-15% of the change in body weight over the length of time

c. Physical exercise alone can be a useful strategy for most people to lose significant weight

d. Significant fluctuations in weight are not associated with an increased risk of cardiovascular disease and all-cause mortality

e. The guidelines issued by various organizations do not vary considerably about the amount of physical activity needed to have a stable weight profile.

The correct statement is "a."

30 to 60 minutes of daily moderate-intensity exercise for five days in a week or vigorous -intensity exercise three times a week is recommended. Considerable variation in guidelines by various organizations exists.

Donnelly, J. E., Blair, S. N., Jakicic, J. M., Manore, M. M., Rankin, J. W., & Smith, B. K. (2009). Appropriate Physical Activity Intervention Strategies for Weight Loss and Prevention of Weight Regain for Adults. Medicine & Science in Sports & Exercise, 41(2), 459-471. doi:10.1249/mss.0b013e3181949333

Question 7.2

Which of the following statements is correct about MET (Metabolic Equivalent), exercise prescription and stress testing?

a. MET is the amount of oxygen consumed or metabolic work done during slow walking, and it is equal to 1 MET

b. Walking at four mph on a level and firm surface is considered 2 METS

c. A minimum exercise prescription should contain five components including frequency, intensity, time, type, and specific precautions

d. Nuclear imaging stress testing can be done easily for all weight ranges

e. None of the above statements is correct.

The correct statement is "c."

The amount of oxygen consumed, or metabolic work done during quiet sitting is considered 1 MET. Light physical activity is < 3 METs. Moderate exercise is 3-6 METS, and vigorous activity is > 6 METs. Standing takes 2 METs.

Pate, R. R. (1995). Physical Activity and Public Health. Jama, 273(5), 402. doi:10.1001/jama.1995.03520290054029

Question 7.3

NEAT is an acronym for non-exercise activity thermogenesis. Which of the following statements is correct about NEAT?

a. Non-exercise related energy expenditure can be up to 2000 kcal.

b. Increasing standing or ambulation time by 2.5 hours every day may result in spending up to 350 kcal additionally

c. Higher NEAT may lead to a decrease in the required amount of heavy exercise target of suggested 300 minutes in a week

d. Climbing stairs can range between 5 to 8 METs of activity

e. All the above statements are correct.

The correct statement is "e."

All the above statements are correct. NEAT's role may establish as more data becomes available. Replacing sedentary behaviors with active lifestyle and activity may help in weight maintenance.

Black AE, Coward WA, Cole TJ, Prentice AM: (1996). Human energy expenditure in affluent

Pharmacology

Question 8.1

Which of the following statements is correct about the use of phentermine in the management of obesity?

a. Phentermine has been in clinical use since 1959 and carries a significant addicting potential.

b. FDA approved phentermine for long-term use up to 36 weeks

c. BMI thresholds are best tools to aid in decision making when prescribing phentermine and the patients should be seen at least every six months.

d. Phentermine belongs to a group of substituted phenethylamines

e. Phentermine does not produce false positive urine drug screen tests

The correct answer is "d."

Phentermine is a controlled medicine and belongs to schedule IV category. It requires a prescription. It does not carry significant addiction potential. FDA has approved it for short-term use. A consensus does not exist about how frequently patients should be followed. Six months seems to be a too long time for follow-up. False positive drug screen tests may occur for amphetamine or methamphetamine while taking phentermine. This may require specific tests to differentiate.

Hendricks, E. J., Rothman, R. B., & Greenway, F. L. (2009). How Physician Obesity Specialists Use Drugs to Treat Obesity. Obesity, 17(9), 1730-1735. doi:10.1038/oby.2009.69

https://www.verywellmind.com/how-long-does-adipex-stay-in-your-system-80217

Question 8.2

Which of the following statements is correct regarding the pharmacology of phentermine?

a. Phentermine base and phentermine hydrochloride have the same potency
b. Phentermine has a half-life of 4 hours.
c. Phentermine is known to have teratogenic effects during pregnancy
d. Titration of the dose of phentermine is not needed
e. Adult obese patients with ADHD may require higher doses of phentermine

The correct answer is "e."

The half-life of phentermine hydrochloride is 7 to 20 hours. Titration of phentermine dose is generally required. It is the observation by some physicians that patients with a diagnosis of ADHD need higher doses of phentermine. There are no teratogenic effects ascribed to phentermine. This drug is not recommended in pregnancy since FDA recommendations in 1979.

Steelman, G. M., & Westman, E. C. Pharmacotherapy. In: Steelman, G. M., & Westman, E. C. (Eds.) Obesity: evaluation and treatment essentials, 2nd Edition. Boca Raton: CRC Press, Taylor & Francis Group Press; 2016, pp.141-145

Question 8.3

A 28-year-old patient with current symptoms of ADHD and chronic diarrhea is started on phentermine. The patient is currently not on any other stimulants. Please select the correct statement.

a. A decreased heart rate is expected

b. Appetite is likely to increase

c. Diarrhea may improve

d. Symptoms of ADHD will increase

e. Intestinal motility will increase

The correct answer is "c."

The adrenergic effect may lead to an increase in heart rate, decrease in appetite, improvement of diarrhea and ADHD symptoms. Intestinal activity may decrease.

Question 8.4

A 35-year-old patient with morbid obesity is prescribed phentermine. She experienced significant insomnia several months after starting the medication. A diagnosis of late-onset insomnia was made. Which of the following statements is <u>not</u> correct regarding managing her symptom?

a. Phentermine dose may be decreased

b. Phentermine may need to be stopped

c. Pindolol may help

d. Benzodiazepines are preferred for this kind of insomnia

e. Trazodone may be tried

The correct answer is "d."

Late-onset insomnia occurs in less than 1 in 1000 patients. It sometimes responds to melatonin, pindolol or trazodone. Benzodiazepines are generally not recommended for this type of insomnia. Early onset insomnia usually responds to pindolol at bedtime.

Question 8.5

A 40-year-old patient with a BMI of 37 is prescribed phentermine. She experiences constipation, lightheadedness, difficulty in micturition and dry mouth. Some of these effects can be explained based on which of the following mechanisms?

a. Cholinergic effects
b. Adrenergic effects
c. Anticholinergic effects
d. Antiadrenergic effects
e. Antidopaminergic effects

The correct answer is "c."

The side effects mentioned above are anticholinergic in nature.

Question 8.6

Which of the following statements is correct about Diethylpropion?

a. Its half-life is similar to phentermine
b. It may be a useful alternate drug for weight loss for people experiencing insomnia with phentermine
c. Its use is considered safe during pregnancy
d. Its use is safe for children below 16 years
e. Diethylpropion cannot be combined with other weight loss medications.

The correct answer is "b."

This medicine has a half-life of 4 to 6 hours. It has been used in patients with the problem of insomnia. This drug is not recommended for pediatric patients and during pregnancy since FDA assigned it category B in 1979. This medicine has been used in combinations with other weight loss drugs.

Cercato, C., Roizenblatt, V. A., Leança, C. C., Segal, A., Filho, A. P., Mancini, M. C., & Halpern, A. (2009). A randomized, double-blind placebo-controlled study of the long-term efficacy and safety of diethylpropion in the treatment of obese subjects. International Journal of Obesity, 33(8), 857-865. doi:10.1038/ijo.2009.124

Question 8.7

Orlistat has been used in the treatment of obesity. Select the correct statement.

a. Orlistat has been proven to be highly successful in clinical practice
b. Its mechanism of action is about inhibition of intestinal lipase to prevent absorption of fat.
c. It can produce oily diarrhea and foul-smelling flatus
d. Its use is not considered safe for children below 16 years
e. b and c are correct

The correct answer is "e."

Due to the side effects, this medicine has not been very successful in clinical practice. It is considered safe for use in the pediatric age group under 16.

Question 8.8

A 28-year-old morbidly obese female is interested in starting Phentermine and Topiramate combination for weight loss. She is normotensive. She has history of renal stones. Which of the following statements is correct about the use of this combination?

a. She needs counseling about risks of birth defects involving craniofacial deformities.
b. She can nurse her baby as these medicines are not excreted in milk.
c. Her chances of having renal stones in future are not increased
d. She may experience dry mouth, and this effect can be due to both Topiramate and phentermine
e. a and d are correct

The correct answer is "e."

Birth defects especially cleft lip and palate may be associated with Topamax use. Safety of these drugs in nursing mothers has not been established. There is some risk of renal stones with use of Topamax. A likely reason for this may be the metabolic acidosis produced by Topamax. Dry mouth can be a troublesome side effect of this combination. Some of the other side effects include paresthesia, oligohydrosis, and hyperkalemia. Topiramate inhibits carbonic anhydrase. Zonisamide (another antiepileptic) has also been reported to cause weight loss.

Question 8.9

Lorcaserin (Belviq®) have been pulled out of market due to which of the following reasons?

a. Risk of GI tumors
b. Risk of Serotonin syndrome
c. Risk of development of cardiac murmurs
d. Addiction risks
e. All the above statements are correct. The correct answer is "a."

This medication was recalled from the marked due to risks of development of various tumors especially involving gastrointestinal system, lung, and breast.

Question 8.10

A 55-year morbidly obese patient with BMI 45 is interested in starting Bupropion/naltrexone combination for weight loss. She has degenerative spine disease and bulging discs. She uses ibuprofen for pain control. Please select the correct statement about the use of this combination.

a. This medication combination is not contraindicated due to concurrent use of NSAIDs.

b. The incremental dose is needed in the first few weeks to avoid some of the side effects

c. Side effect of nausea is generally due to naltrexone component

d. This drug does not fall in the category of controlled substances as classified by DEA

e. All the above statements are correct

The correct answer is "e."

Bupropion is an antidepressant and naltrexone is an opioid receptor antagonist. This combination cannot be used if patient is taking narcotic medications. However, it can be used if NSAIDs are prescribed for pain control. An incremental dose of the combination is recommended to avoid some of the side effects. Nausea occurs due to naltrexone component. This drug is not classified as a controlled medicine.

Greenway, F. L., Dunayevich, E., Tollefson, G., Erickson, J., Guttadauria, M., Fujioka, K., & Cowley, M. A. (2009). Comparison of Combined Bupropion and Naltrexone Therapy for Obesity with Monotherapy and Placebo. The Journal of Clinical Endocrinology & Metabolism, 94(12), 4898-4906. doi:10.1210/jc.2009-1350

Question 8.11

Topiramate has been used in combination with phentermine or alone in obesity management for many years. Which of the following statements is correct about the use of this medication?

a. This medication is found to be useful in controlling binge eating and weight gain due to antidepressant medication use.

b. FDA has not approved this medication for weight loss, so its use for this condition is regarded as "Off-label." Patients need to be counseled about this.

c. Neurologic symptoms are due to its weak inhibition of carbonic anhydrase activity

d. Acute closed-angle Glaucoma is an idiosyncratic reaction of topiramate and should be urgently addressed with appropriate referral and stopping the medication.

e. All the above statements are correct

The correct answer is "e."

Topiramate is a commonly used off-label drug for weight loss. It is found to be useful for controlling hunger symptoms. It helps reduce craving for carbohydrates and sweets. Beneficial effects are observed in disorders like binge eating and drug-induced weight gain after use of antidepressants. Acute closed angle glaucoma can precipitate with topiramate use in patients with narrow angles. The condition requires emergent attention. It can result in blindness if not addressed promptly.

Atrup A, Caterrson I, Zelissen P, Guy-Grand B, Carruba M, Levy B, et al. (2004). Topiramate long-term maintenance of weight loss induced by a low-calorie diet in obese subjects Obes Res 12,1658-1669

Question 8.12

Which of the following statements is correct about Liraglutide?

a. It is a GLP-1 receptor agonist
b. It is a GLP-1 receptor antagonist
c. It decreases insulin release
d. It increases glucagon release
e. It increases food intake and promotes weight gain

The correct answer is "a."

Liraglutide is a long-acting GLP-1 analog. This activates the GLP-1 receptor in the pancreatic islet cells. It increases insulin release and lowers glucagon secretion. This drug reduces food intake and promotes weight loss. This may also increase the risk of medullary thyroid neoplasm and pancreatitis.

Gorgojo-Martínez, J. J., Feo-Ortega, G., & Serrano-Moreno, C. (2016). Effectiveness and tolerability of liraglutide in patients with type 2 diabetes mellitus and obesity after bariatric surgery. Surgery for Obesity and Related Diseases, 12(10), 1856-1863. doi: 10.1016/j.soard.2016.02.013

Question 8.13

Which of the following statements is correct about pharmacological effects of Liraglutide?

a. It increases gastric emptying
b. It raises blood sugar
c. It decreases satiety
d. It decreases gastric emptying
e. It does not affect gastric emptying

The correct answer is "d."

Liraglutide is a GLP -1 agonist. It decreases gastric emptying time, reduces hunger, decreases caloric intake and blood sugar. These effects promote weight loss.

Niswender, K., Pi-Sunyer, X., Buse, J., Jensen, K. H., Toft, A. D., Russell-Jones, D., & Zinman, B. (2012). Weight change with liraglutide and comparator therapies: an analysis of seven phase 3 trials from the liraglutide diabetes development programme. Diabetes, Obesity and Metabolism, 15(1), 42-54. doi:10.1111/j.1463-1326.2012. 01673.x

Question 8.14

A 39-year-old woman with BMI of 37, is seen in a Bariatric office. She describes premenstrual craving for chocolates, sugars, and carbohydrates. She has gained 20 pounds in the last three months. Her fat distribution is predominantly in pelvic area and thighs. Some edema of legs is noted as well. She has several high blood pressure readings, and family doctor is considering starting some antihypertensive medication. Appropriate nutritional counseling was done. Which of the following medications can be a cost-effective and useful option for her to reduce symptoms of food craving in addition to help control blood pressure and edema?

a. Spironolactone hydrochlorothiazide combination
b. Metoprolol
c. Hydralazine
d. Nafidipine
e. Captopril.

The correct answer is "a"

Some experienced authors have cited spironolactone /hydrochlorothiazide combination (25 mg dose for each) may be helpful in preventing some of the premenstrual symptoms of craving for sweets and carbohydrates in addition to treating high blood pressure and edema. This scenario highlights the importance of keeping patient's overall clinical picture in mind as multiple conditions can be addressed with a medication or a combination. Edema is common in obese patients. Clinicians need to differentiate edema from lipedema. The latter condition may respond to physical therapy and compression dressings. It may also need surgical intervention.

Steelman, G. M., & Westman, E. C. Pharmacotherapy. In: Steelman, G. M., & Westman, E. C. (Eds.) Obesity: evaluation and treatment essentials, 2nd Edition. Boca Raton: CRC Press, Taylor & Francis Group Press; 2016, pp.157

Question 8.15

A 37-year-old woman with BMI of 31 is prescribed liraglutide (Saxenda®) *. She is also known to have DM 2. A few months later she presents with severe upper abdominal pain along with nausea and vomiting. She has a white cell count of 14.3. Blood sugar is 280mg /dl, liver functions are normal, and urine analysis is in the normal range. Her blood sugars have not been very well controlled in the last few months. Which of the following statements is correct regarding her clinical condition?

a. GERD (gastroesophageal reflux disease) is a more likely diagnosis
b. Colitis is a common side effect of liraglutide
c. A CT scan of the abdomen may show stranding in retrogastric and duodenal C area
d. Ultrasound of the abdomen may not be helpful
e. None of the above statements is true

The correct answer is "c."

Please see explanation with Question 16

*Saxenda® is a registered trademark of Novo Nordisk A/S

Question 8.16

Patient in the above question was discharged later when her additional workup was found to be negative. She follows with her family doctor a few days later. She is considered for starting some additional medication to control diabetes. Which of the following statements is correct?

a. Insulin and liraglutide combination can be an option
b. Liraglutide dose should not be increased to have better control of diabetes
c. Liraglutide is not very cost effective for most patients
d. It is only available as an injection
e. All above statements are correct

The correct answer is "e."

Statements “a” to “d” are correct. Patients on Liraglutide carry an increased risk of developing pancreatitis and gallstones. Any acute upper abdominal pain needs evaluation with these diagnoses in mind. A CT scan study may show changes related to pancreatitis with stranding. Sonogram of the gallbladder may show stones or sludge.

Need Help Taking Off Excess Weight and Keeping It Off? (n.d.). Retrieved January 02, 2018, from https://www.saxenda.com/

Question 8.17

A 30-year-old morbidly obese male was diagnosed with HIV infection. Antiretroviral therapy was started with zidovudine. He is given handouts and links to the information about side effects of HIV medications. At his next family doctor's office visit, he asks several questions from his provider. Please select the correct statement.

a. He has decreased risk of hyperglycemia
b. He is less likely to have dyslipidemia
c. His visceral fat is likely to increase
d. He is less likely to develop lipodystrophy
e. Increased subcutaneous adiposity

The correct answer is "c."

Older HIV medications have led to lipodystrophy in many patients. Newer medications do not have this side effect.

"Factsheet Lipodystrophy." HIV & AIDS Information, www.aidsmap.com/Lipodystrophy/page/1045065/.

Question 8.18

A 27-year-old morbidly obese female is diagnosed with polycystic ovarian syndrome (PCOS) and insulin resistance. Her liver functions are abnormal. Lab work show AST and ALT both raised by 30% from base values. She takes tricyclic antidepressants regularly. She is recently found to be HIV positive and considering antiretroviral therapy. She has recently joined a weight loss program. While taking history, it is also found that her father had colon cancer at the age of 45 and mother developed breast cancer at the age of 39 years. Her lab work shows slightly raised insulin levels. Which of the following medications may be a useful choice for her considering her existing list of multiple diagnoses and risk factors?

a. Phentermine

b. Sucralfate

c. Metformin

d. Naltrexone/bupropion combination

e. Topiramate

The correct answer is "c."

Metformin is considered useful for insulin resistance, fatty liver, and PCOS. It may be helpful in preventing some of the weight-related complications with use of anti retroviral medications. and some antidepressants. Another potential benefit exists in colon cancer prevention.

Johnson, N P. “Metformin Use in Women with Polycystic Ovary Syndrome.” Annals of Translational Medicine., U.S. National Library of Medicine, June 2014, www.ncbi.nlm.nih.gov/pubmed/25333031.

Question 8.19

A 32-year-old morbidly obese female is followed in a bariatric program. She carries a BMI of 49. She has several stressors in life, and the recent loss of her mother has made her very depressed. She sees a counselor. A consideration is made by her family physician to start some antidepressant. Please select the medication which can be relatively weight neutral.

a. Imipramine
b. Paroxetine
c. Fluoxetine
d. Amitriptyline
e. Doxepin

The correct answer is "c."

Fluoxetine seems to be a better choice among the stated medications due to less weight gaining potential.

Hasnain, Mehrul, et al. “Weight Gain and Glucose Dysregulation with Second-Generation Antipsychotics and Antidepressants: A Review for Primary Care Physicians.” Postgraduate Medicine, vol. 124, no. 4, 2012, pp. 154–167., doi:10.3810/pgm.2012.07.2577.

Question 8.20

A 40-year-old male with BMI 37 follows a weight loss program. He has a history of depression for many years. Lately due to loss of job, depression has become worse. He smokes a pack daily for the last eight years. Discussion between the counselor, bariatrician and family doctor in the multidisciplinary meeting takes place. Currently, he is on doxepin. Concerns are raised about the weight gaining potential of the medication. Reasonable choice for his symptoms of depression could be which one of the following medications?

a. Imipramine
b. Paroxetine
c. Bupropion
d. Amitriptyline
e. Doxepin

The correct answer is "c."

Bupropion seems to be a reasonable choice for him. It may be beneficial for control of depression symptoms along with help in quitting smoking. It may also help losing weight. Bupropion in combination with naltrexone is an approved weight loss medication.

Question 8.21

A 30-year-old female with BMI 33 underwent sleeve gastrectomy procedure a couple of years ago. She has also undergone cholecystectomy and tubal ligation. She has lost 55 pounds of weight since surgery. She has started gaining weight for the last few months. She craves for chips and crackers in the evenings. She had severe anxiety and had developed panic attacks a few times in the recent months. She also has a history of migraines. Currently, she gets severe headaches which are affecting her quality of life. She follows a neurologist. Which of the following medications may help improve her symptoms?

a. Phentermine

b. Paroxetine

c. Bupropion

d. Topiramate

e. Bupropion and naltrexone combination

The correct answer is "d."

Here topiramate may be a better choice. It may address her issues of headaches and help improve cravings for starches. Phentermine should be avoided in her case due to anxiety and panic attacks. Use of Topamax for weight loss remains off-label. Any female with childbearing potential needs to be educated about pregnancy related risks with its use.

Question 8.22

Please select the medication which has the most potential of weight gain.

a. Clozapine
b. Trazodone
c. Benzodiazepines
d. Amisulpride
e. Melatonin

The correct answer is "a."

In this list of sedatives, clozapine has the most potential of weight gain.

Question 8.23

A 34-year-old lady is seeking help to lose weight in a weight loss program. Her medical reconciliation reveals methylphenidate (Ritalin®) prescribed for ADHD. She also takes medications for hypertension. Her blood pressure fluctuates. She has anxiety issues at times. She is given distinct options. She is interested in starting phentermine/topiramate combination to help control cravings for food. Please select the correct statement.

a. Phentermine and methylphenidate have similar potential of producing dependence

b. Both medicines can be used safely together

c. Methylphenidate and phentermine should be avoided together as her blood pressure control may be affected

d. The patient may see more anxiety issues due to the stimulant nature of both medications if used simultaneously

e. "c" and "d" are correct

The correct answer is "e."

Phentermine is schedule IV, and methylphenidate is schedule II drug. Later has more potential for dependence. Concurrent use in her case should be avoided for reasons of stimulant nature and potential effect on her blood pressure.

Question 8.24

Topiramate /phentermine combination is started for a morbidly obese patient to help control cravings for sweets and carbs. One week after starting the treatment she felt blurry vision and discomfort in eyes. She calls her physician's office. The provider suspects development of acute glaucoma. An emergency referral is arranged to see an ophthalmologist. Please select the correct statement about her clinical condition.

a. Her glaucoma is likely to be an open angle glaucoma
b. Drainage channels for aqueous humor in trabecular meshwork between iris and cornea are blocked
c. A defect in the ciliary body due to edema and displacement leading to closing the angle between iris and cornea is a likely reason
d. Alkaline phosphatase is a key enzyme in controlling the aqueous humor production
e. Topiramate increase carbonic anhydrase production

The correct answer is "c."

Acute narrow-angle glaucoma is reported as a complication with use of some of the weight loss medications including topiramate. It requires urgent evaluation and treatment. Blindness may result if a delay in treatment occurs. Topiramate is a weak inhibitor of carbonic anhydrase. This enzyme is involved in aqueous humor production.

Question 8.25

A 52-year-old female is noted to have gained 20 pounds at her annual physical with her primary care physician. She has several medical problems. She has a long of list of medications. Some of the medications were started in the past year. At medical reconciliation, she is found to be taking metoprolol for hypertension, glipizide /metformin for diabetes, Gabapentin for chronic pain issues. She has started taking bupropion for depression a few months back. Please select the correct statement.

a. Both Metoprolol and bupropion can cause weight gain
b. Both Metformin and Gabapentin can cause weight gain
c. Both Glipizide and bupropion can cause weight gain
d. Both Metformin and bupropion can cause weight gain
e. Both Metformin and metoprolol can cause weight gain
f. Both Metoprolol and glipizide can cause weight gain

The correct answer is "f."

Metoprolol, glipizide, gabapentin can cause weight gain.

Question 8.26

Which of the following weight loss medication should not be used in patients with suicidal ideations?

a. Phentermine topiramate combination
b. Orlistat
c. Naltrexone HCL and bupropion combination
d. Liraglutide
e. None of the above medications is associated with suicidal ideation
f. Options a, c, and d

The correct answer is "f."

Phentermine topiramate combination, naltrexone bupropion combination and liraglutide should be avoided in patient with suicidal ideations.

https://www.drugs.com/disease-interactions/liraglutide,victoza.html

https://www.rxlist.com/contrave-drug.htm#warnings

Question 8.27

A 45-year-old female with BMI of 37 is started on Topiramate (off label) to help control cravings for sweets and carbohydrates. As part of follow up, a panel of labs is requested after a couple of months of use. Which of the following metabolic side effects is anticipated?

a. Metabolic acidosis
b. Metabolic alkalosis
c. Respiratory acidosis
d. Respiratory alkalosis

Correct answer is "a."

Topiramate inhibits carbonic anhydrase, and it may lead to renal bicarbonate loss and development of metabolic acidosis.

Questions 8.28

Fatty liver disease management can be challenging. Please select the correct statement.

a. GLP1 agonists have an indirect beneficial effect on fatty liver by causing weight loss
b. Pioglitazone can help prevent the progression of fibrosis in fatty liver disease
c. Pioglitazone can precipitate CHF
d. 10 percent weight loss may improve NASH by 80%
e. All above statements are correct.

Correct answer is “e.”

Pioglitazone belongs to thiazolidinedione class. It improves the sensitivity of insulin. Its side effects include bladder carcinoma, hypoglycemia, CHF, and osteoporosis. Contraindications include pregnancy and breast feeding.

Question 8.29

Glomerular filtration rate remains important in calculating doses of many pharmacological agents. Which of the following statements is correct about the estimated glomerular filtration rate in patients after bariatric surgery?

a. In post-bariatric surgery cases, estimated glomerular filtration rate (GFR) remains as one of most reliable methods of renal function assessment.
b. Estimated GFR does not depend on creatinine
c. Estimated GFR is likely to decrease in post-bariatric patients due to loss of muscle mass
d. Estimated GFR does not take into account the surface area of the patient
e. In post-bariatric surgery patients, estimated GFR may increase without real improvement of renal function

The correct answer is "e."

This interesting fact is derived from several observations. After bariatric surgery patients lose some muscle mass. GFR data tables are obtained from patients who are not obese and decreased body surface area after losing weight is not adjusted in GFR calculations. This issue may lead to incorrect estimations of GFR. Some of the equations used in the assessment of GFR include CKD-EPI, MDRD, and Cockcroft-Gault. The later one incorporates lean body mass adjustments.

Editorial Board. (2016). Surgery for Obesity and Related Diseases, 12(1), I-Ii. doi:10.1016/s1550-7289(15)01029-1

Question 8.30

Several medications are known to affect lipid and carbohydrate metabolism. Which of the following medications may lead to hyperglycemia, lipid disorder, decreased subcutaneous fat and more visceral fat accumulation?

a. Loop diuretics
b. Proton pump inhibitors
c. Antiretroviral therapy
d. Cephalosporins
e. Chronic coumadin use

The correct answer is "c."

Antiretroviral therapy is noted to have stated side effects. Metformin may help in preventing some of these effects.

Question 8.31

In evaluating an obese patient, it may be useful to have an assessment of fat-free mass and lean body mass. These calculations remain important in determining doses of some medications and nutritional goals. Please select the correct statement.

a. Lean body mass is total body mass minus fatty tissues. In a nonobese person it is generally 75% of total body mass.
b. Fat-free mass is total body mass minus total body fat.
c. Lean body mass differs from the fat free mass by approximately 5%
d. Fat-free mass can be measured with techniques like dual-energy x-ray absorptiometry (DXA) scan or bioelectrical impedance (BIA)
e. All the above statements are correct.

The correct answer is "e."

Fat-free mass is the sum of water, minerals, protein, and glycogen of body. On the other hand, lean body mass is the sum of water, mineral, protein, glycogen, fat in organs, bone marrow, and CNS.

Question 8.32

A 37-year-old lady had biliopancreatic diversion procedure with duodenal switch for super morbid obesity, eight years ago. She is seen in her family doctor's office for annual physical examination. She is complaining of bruises and heavy periods. She takes over the counter vitamins. Which of the following statements is correct about her clinical condition?

a. One of the group B water-soluble vitamin deficiencies could be a probable cause

b. Fat soluble vitamin deficiencies are infrequently seen

c. Vitamin E deficiency is likely reasons for her symptoms.

d. Vitamin K deficiency is seen in more than 50 % of patients with biliopancreatic diversion.

e. Vitamin K supplements are not helpful

The correct answer is "d."

Biliopancreatic diversion has a high metabolic impact due to significant malabsorption. Patients are vulnerable to develop multiple nutritional deficiencies. Fat-soluble vitamins need special attention. Fat soluble vitamin are A, D, E and K.

Fujioka, K., Dibaise, J. K., & Martindale, R. G. (2011). Nutrition and Metabolic Complications After Bariatric Surgery and Their Treatment. Journal of Parenteral and Enteral Nutrition, 35(5_suppl). doi:10.1177/0148607111413600

Question 8.33

A 45-year-old lady presents to the bariatric office. She underwent Roux-en-Y gastric bypass 12 years ago. She has a history of marginal ulcers. She continues to be a smoker. Her current list of medications includes Pantoprazole, Fluoxetine, Trazodone, Pepto-Bismol, Iron, Calcium, and vitamin D. Her bariatric surgeon notes blackish tongue. Which of the following statements is correct?

a. Iron deficiency is suspected.
b. The color change of tongue is likely related to her smoking
c. Bismuth sulfide is the likely reason for her black tongue
d. This condition is suggestive of acanthosis nigricans.
e. Antidepressant medications on her list are likely to cause of her black tongue.

The correct answer is "c."

Bismuth component of Pepto-Bismol combines with sulfur in saliva generating bismuth sulfide. This compound gives black color to the tongue. It is considered harmless and stays for a brief period. Acanthosis nigricans does not involve tongue. It involves armpits, groins, skin of back of neck, and anogenital region.

Why does Pepto-Bismol sometimes darken the tongue/stool and how long does it last? (n.d.). Retrieved December 29,

2017, from http://www.pepto-bismol.com/en-us/faq/black-stool-black-tongue

Question 8.34
A 43-year-old female presents with numbness and tingling in the hands and feet. She had Roux-en-Y gastric bypass surgery 11 years ago. Her examination reveals nystagmus and some degree of confusion. Which of the following statements is correct about her clinical condition?

a. Wernicke's encephalopathy is a likely possibility
b. Absorption of thiamine is affected due to less food intake, less acid, and exclusion of duodenum
c. Concurrent B12 deficiency may also add to neural symptoms
d. Prompt treatment of the condition is needed to prevent long-term sequelae
e. All the above statements are correct

The correct answer is "e."

All the factors stated in option "b" can contribute to B1 (thiamine) deficiency. Physicians should have a high index of suspicion in dealing with any vulnerable patient. Prompt treatment can prevent long-term sequelae of Wernicke's encephalopathy. Thiamine deficiency can also lead to Beriberi. It is recognized in two forms including wet and dry types. Post gastric bypass patients with prolonged nausea and vomiting should be checked for the deficiency of B1. B12 deficiency should also be considered in patients with malabsorptive procedures.

John, Seeniann, and Carl Hoegerl. "Nutritional Deficiencies After Gastric Bypass Surgery." The Journal of the American Osteopathic Association, American Osteopathic Association, 1 Nov. 2009, jaoa.org/article.aspx?articleid=2093757.

Question 8.35

A 33-year-old female is admitted with diarrhea and skin lesions in the form of desquamating and peeling rash at extremities and perioral areas for the last several weeks. She had Roux-en-Y gastric bypass eight years ago. She consumes alcohol on a regular basis. Her vital signs were stable. Systemic examination was otherwise normal. Her lab work showed mild anemia and mild abnormality of liver enzymes. Zinc level was 0.25 μg/mL (0.66–1.10 μg/mL). Which of the following statements is <u>not</u> correct about Zinc deficiency in Bariatric patients?

a. Zinc deficiency is suspected in the setting of post gastric bypass patients with a history of diarrhea and peeling skin rash

b. The primary absorption of zinc occurs in Jejunum

c. Niacin deficiency may have similar symptoms.

d. Most zinc deficiency cases require IV replacement of zinc.

e. Zinc sulfate, zinc gluconate, and Zinc acetate have been used for oral replacement

The correct answer is "d."

Duodenum and proximal jejunum are the primary sites for the absorption of zinc. Patients who had a duodenal switch or Roux-en-Y gastric bypass operation, are more vulnerable to zinc deficiency. Diarrhea, dermatitis, poor wound healing, cognitive dysfunction, and immune dysfunction are related clinical features. Most cases can be treated with oral zinc supplements.

Shahsavari, D., Ahmed, Z., Karikkineth, A., Williams, R., & Zigel, C. (2014). Zinc-deficiency acrodermatitis in a patient with chronic alcoholism and gastric bypass: a case report. Journal of Community Hospital Internal Medicine Perspectives, 4(3), 24707. doi:10.3402/jchimp. v4.24707

Question 8.36

A 35-year-old patient had Roux-en-Y Gastric bypass five years ago. She presents with symptoms of craving for ice and nonfood items including paper, dirt, clay, cornstarch, and paints. She feels shortness of breath on exertion. On examination, she has pallor of conjunctiva. Her health provider also notes dark circles under the eyes and spoon-shaped nails. She appears lethargic. Which of the following statements is correct about her clinical condition?

a. B12 and folic acid deficiency is suspected

b. Calcium and vitamin D deficiency is suspected.

c. Copper, Zinc deficiency is suspected

d. Iron deficiency is suspected

The correct answer is "d."

Symptoms mentioned here are suggestive of Iron deficiency. These may typically be seen in patients who had malabsorptive bariatric procedures. These include Roux-en-Y gastric bypass and duodenal switch procedures. Iron deficiency can be severe in females who have heavy periods and those who are not taking oral iron supplements regularly.

Love, A. L., & Billett, H. H. (2008). Obesity, bariatric surgery, and iron deficiency: True, and related. American Journal of Hematology, 83(5), 403-409. DOI: 10.1002/ajh.21106

Question 8.37

A 32-year-old female with BMI of 48, is exploring bariatric surgery options. She is referred to a Bariatrician for a pre-operative assessment. She is interested in Roux-en-Y gastric bypass. A discussion was done about nutritional and vitamin deficiencies. The patient is especially counseled about the risks of various vitamin and micronutrient deficiencies after surgery. Which of the following statements is true regarding B12 deficiency?

a. Prevalence of B12 deficiency is <u>not</u> high in patients who take proton pump inhibitors

b. Serum B12 level is always adequate to identify B12 deficiency

c. Elevated Methylmalonic acid (MMA) level may be a more reliable indicator of B12 status

d. Increase serum homocysteine, and normal MMA level indicates a B12 deficiency

e. None of the above statements is true

The correct answer is "c."

Elevated Methylmalonic acid MMA has been found to be more reliable in diagnosing B12 deficiency. This test may help distinguish folic acid deficiency. Homocysteine level can be elevated in both B12 and Folic acid deficiencies.

Parrott J, Frank L, Guidelines for the Surgical Weight Loss Patient 2016 Update: Micronutrients Surg Obes Relat Dis 2017;13:727–741.

Question 8.38

A 40-year-old patient who had Roux-en-Y gastric bypass a few years ago presents to the emergency room. She had a history of recurrent marginal ulcers. Her current symptoms include persistent nausea and vomiting for the last two weeks with progressive worsening. She appears to have developed ataxia, nystagmus, confusion, and numbness. Which of the following statements is true?

a. MRI of the brain is unlikely to show increased T2 changes in thalamus, hypothalamus, enhancement of bilateral mammillary bodies and midline cerebellum

b. The deficiency is expected from a vitamin absorbed mainly in the terminal ileum

c. Her symptoms will improve with high doses of vitamin B12

d. A similar condition may be seen in chronic alcoholics

e. Her symptoms are likely to improve with high doses of vitamin D

The correct answer is "d."

Ataxia, nystagmus, and confusion with numbness can develop with B1 deficiency. This condition can be seen in alcoholics as well. Wernicke's encephalopathy needs prompt treatment with intravenous B1 administration to prevent long-term neurological sequelae. MRI scan of the brain may show changes in hypothalamus, thalamus, and related areas. In this scenario vitamin D has no role.

Question 8.39

Regarding patient stated in the previous question select the correct statement

a. The patient is more likely to be a male

b. The human body has a store of the expected deficient nutrient for several months

c. Exposure of skin to sunlight help to prevent this disorder

d. Symptoms are reversible in almost all patients with adequate and timely replacement of deficient nutrient

e. As compared to a CT scan, MRI scan is more likely to hint about CNS abnormalities in this disorder

The correct answer is "e."

Condition appears to be more common in the females. Human body does not have large stores of B1. Patient with history of nausea or vomiting are more vulnerable to have B1 deficiency. Sunlight helps in production of vitamin D and not of vitamin B1. MRI scan is considered more sensitive in picking CNS abnormalities seen in Wernicke's encephalopathy.

Alias T, Hoof P, Lee M, Davis D. Wernicke's encephalopathy after conversion from sleeve gastrectomy to gastric bypass. Surgery For Obesity and Related Disease. 2016; 12:89-91

Question 8.40

Select the correct statement about recommended minimum daily intake of Vitamin D3 (Cholecalciferol) after bariatric surgery.

a. 400 international units

b. 800 international units

c. 100 international units

d. 3000 international units

The correct answer is "d."

A dose of 3000 IU to 50000 IU one to three times weekly is recommended by ASMBS, TOS and AACE.

Question 8.41

The recommended dose of daily calcium after bariatric surgery is

a. 500 mg

b. 1000 mg

c. 1200-1500 mg, and 1800-2400 mg after duodenal switch procedure.

d. 5000 mg

The correct answer is "c."

Question 8.42

Recommended daily dose of elemental Iron after bariatric surgery is

a. 10 mg

b. 45-60 mg

c. 100 mg

d. 500 mg

The correct answer is "b."

Parrott, J., Frank, L., Rabena, R., Craggs-Dino, L., Isom, K. A., & Greiman, L. (2017). American Society for Metabolic and Bariatric Surgery Integrated Health Nutritional Guidelines for the Surgical Weight Loss Patient 2016 Update: Micronutrients. Surgery for Obesity and Related Diseases, 13(5), 727-741. doi: 10.1016/j.soard.2016.12.018

Question 8.43

A female with a history of sleeve gastrectomy is seen on a follow-up visit in her primary care physician's office. Recent lab work is also available. Her hemoglobin is 9.5. Serum Iron and ferritin levels are low. She is prescribed oral iron therapy. Which of the following vitamins given concurrently can help improve iron absorption?

a. Vitamin A
b. Vitamin B2
c. Vitamin C
d. Vitamin D
e. Vitamin K

The correct answer is "c."

Vitamin C helps keep the ferric irons chelated at acid pH. It is more soluble at a high pH of the duodenum. Vitamin C is especially helpful in the absorption of iron from vegetable meals.

Question 8.44

A 42-year-old morbidly obese female with problems of DM2, HTN, and Hyperlipidemia opts for Roux-en-Y gastric bypass surgery for weight loss. Her pre-operative BMI was 52. She has a couple of C-Sections in past. Preoperative sonogram of the abdomen shows fatty liver. Gallbladder was normal. She lost about 45 pounds in four months after her bariatric procedure. She presents in the emergency with an acute right upper quadrant abdominal pain. She is currently taking medications for HTN, diabetes, oral multivitamins, and iron. She has a WBC count of 13.1, K 3.8, AST 101, ALT 92, and total bilirubin is 3.7 with a direct bilirubin level of 2.1. Please select the correct statement.

a. Rapid weight loss has no contribution to the development of her acute condition
b. Gallbladder disorder is an unlikely pathology
c. An ultrasound of right upper quadrant will be an initial investigation of choice in her case
d. Common bile duct dilates (CBD) in all cases of gastric bypass even if they do not have common bile duct stones.
e. An ERCP (endoscopic retrograde cholangiopancreatography) through the mouth can resolve her issue

The correct answer is "c."

Question 8.45

In relation to prevention and management of the problem stated in the above question, select the correct statement

a. Calcium chloride has been proven to prevent the formation of gallstones
b. Occurrence of cholesterol and bile pigment gallstones can be completely prevented with the use of bile acid products
c. Ursodeoxycholic acid is a cholesterol-lowering agent
d. Removal of the gallbladder is practiced by most surgeons to prevent gallstone complications following gastric bypass surgery
e. Patient may likely need cholecystectomy and an ERCP (endoscopic retrograde cholangiopancreatography) through the excluded stomach with operative access.

The correct answer is "e."

Gallstones and acute gallbladder condition may occur at a slightly higher frequency following rapid weight loss, especially after bariatric surgical procedures. Mobilization of cholesterol and other lipids may contribute to the development of this condition. Prophylactic removal of an otherwise normal gallbladder is not a universally accepted option. Studies have shown the reduction of gallstone incidence by approximately thirty percent with use of bile acid products following bariatric surgery. The incidence of gallstone formation is higher in initial 6 months following bariatric surgery. It has also been noted that compliance for bile acid products like ursodeoxycholic acid is poor to fair in general due to side effects. Calcium chloride may help prevent formation of renal oxalate stones. Renal stone may form at higher frequency after gastric bypass due to altered calcium and fatty acid metabolism due to malabsorption component of gastric bypass. Ultrasound is more sensitive in picking gallstones. CT scan can miss some radiolucent stones. CBD dilatation is seen in patients who have previous cholecystectomy. Up to 6mm size is considered normal. Stones in CBD can lead to common bile duct dilatation. MRI scan can be helpful to identify CBD stones.

Sattaratnamai, A., et al. "Gallstone Formation and Subsequent Cholecystectomy after Bariatric Surgery: A Systematic Review." Hpb, vol. 18, 2016, doi:10.1016/j.hpb.2016.03.375.

Question 8.46

Select the correct statement about vitamin D

a. Vitamin D is found in most naturally occurring foods
b. Vitamin D3 is produced in the skin with ultraviolet light exposure by a non-enzymatic process
c. D2 is a synthetic form (ergocalciferol)
d. All the above statements are correct.

Correct answer is "b."
Most natural foods are deficient in vitamin D. Even Milk does not contain vitamin D and is added to milk by dairy industry. Natural sunlight is a good source of vitamin D. Vitamin D3 is the form produced in skin with ultraviolet light exposure. Ability of skin to produce D3 decreases significantly beyond the age of 70. Obese patients are at higher risk of vitamin D deficiency. It can lead to secondary changes including hypocalcemia, secondary hyperparathyroidism, phosphaturia, and osteoporosis. 3000 to 6000 IU of D3 daily is recommended to treat vitamin D deficiency. 50,000 IU of D2 (ergocalciferol) one to three times a week can also be used to

treat vitamin D deficiency. Ergocalciferol (D2) is found in mushrooms and other plant resources.

Question 8.47

A 47-year-old female who is 5 years out from gastric bypass surgery for morbid obesity, presents with neurological symptoms affecting lower extremities. Physical examination reveals pallor of conjunctiva. She is also noted to have mild ataxia. Blood work shows anemia of microcytic type. Her hemoglobin is 9.2 and white cell count is 3700. Neutrophils are only 11%. She is in process of changing her health insurance plan and cannot afford co-pay for any additional tests. Her health care provider starts oral iron therapy with a clinical suspicion of iron deficiency. She does not take any other vitamins regularly. Patient is followed in 6 weeks. Her anemia seems not to be improving. Her symptoms of ataxia are worsened. Please select the correct statement regarding her clinical condition.

a. Her iron dose should be increased
b. She should continue with Iron with a B12 shot in the office
c. Selenium deficiency should be suspected
d. Zinc deficiency may be the reason for her symptoms
e. Copper deficiency should be suspected

Correct answer is "e."

Copper deficiency could be a reason. Copper level should be checked in her case. Copper is absorbed in stomach and duodenum. Patients with a history of gastric bypass surgery are vulnerable to copper deficiency. Copper deficiency in malabsorptive procedures like Roux-en-Y gastric bypass and duodenal switch operations is rare but a well-documented condition.

Question 8.48

A patient with history of gastric bypass 12 years ago is diagnosed with copper deficiency. She takes iron for anemia and low ferritin levels. She has received iron infusions in the past. She takes Zinc regularly as well for low Zinc levels. Medical reconciliation reveals that she takes a multivitamin preparation containing molybdenum and selenium. She is advised to take copper sulphate preparation for the copper deficiency. Which of the following supplements can conflict with the absorption of copper?

a. Iron
b. Zinc
c. Selenium
d. Molybdenum

Correct answer is "b."

Zinc and Copper compete for absorption. Concurrent ingestion of Zinc for a long period of time can lead to copper deficiency. This can result in myelopathy.

https://www.uptodate.com/contents/copper-deficiency-myeloneuropathy?search=copper%20deficiency&source=sear

ch_result&selectedTitle=1~60&usage_type=default&display_rank=1

Question 8.49

A post gastric bypass patient who is currently a smoker presents with pain in epigastric area. She smokes a pack daily. She has developed marginal ulcers in the past and had one incidence of marginal ulcer perforation requiring laparoscopic repair. An attempt to quit smoking in past caused her to gain weight. Bariatric surgeon is working closely with family physician to help her stop smoking. A decision is made to check her biochemistry randomly for compliance for nonsmoking. Please select the correct statement.

a. Nicotine half-life is about 0.5 to 3 hours and for Continine it is about 16 to 19 hours
b. Tobacco cigarette and "vaping" e-cigarettes produce similar level of continine
c. Gastric bypass status does not alter the pharmacokinetics or dynamics of nicotine
d. Stopping smoking frequently results in weight gain
e. All above statements are correct

Correct answer is "e."

Statements (a) to (d) are correct. Continine level is the preferred test to check for tobacco use and compliance for nonsmoking. Some of the other short-lived metabolites useful to check for smoking status include anabasine and nornicotine. Nicotine does carry a suppressant effect on appetite. Smoking increases the risk of developing and non-healing of marginal ulcers.

Question 8.50

A 19-year-old girl is diagnosed with polycystic ovaries. She has a BMI of 39. She has irregular periods. Lab work shows high insulin levels suggestive of insulin resistance. She is started on metformin. She also sees a nutritionist and a counselor. She is told about the possibility of use of this medication on long-term basis. She will be prone to have which of the following deficiencies with long-term use of metformin.?

a. Vitamin B1

b. Vitamin B2

c. Vitamin B6

d. Vitamin B12

e. None of the above vitamin deficiency is associated with long-term use of metformin

The correct answer is "d."

Pediatric Obesity—Assessment, Treatment, and Prevention ... academic.oup.com/jcem/article/102/3/709/2965084.

Question 8.51

A 16-year-old girl is started on prescription strength Orlistat to help lose weight. She is also diagnosed with hypothyroidism and takes levothyroxine. She lost 12 pounds in the last 4 months. Her family is very supportive. She has made dietary changes and goes to gym regularly. She presents in the emergency department with severe right upper quadrant pain. Please select to correct statement.

a. Liver functions need to be monitored
b. Biliary stones can form with the use of orlistat
c. Levothyroxine level may drop with use of orlistat
d. Renal function impairment may happen
e. All the above statements are correct

The correct answer is "e."

All the statements from “a” to “d” are correct.

Pediatric Obesity—Assessment, Treatment, and Prevention ... academic.oup.com/jcem/article/102/3/709/2965084.

Question 8.52

A 19-year-old girl is found to have insulin resistance. Her BMI is 43. Her insulin level is in range of 35 to 40. She is started on metformin 500 mg orally twice daily. After two day she calls the office complaining of abdominal pain and diarrhea. Please select to correct statement about her condition.

a. Switching to slow-release preparation of metformin may not be helpful
b. Clostridium Difficile infections are common after metformin use
c. Metformin causes bowel ischemia leading to diarrhea and pain
d. Genetic variation may exist regarding side effects and tolerance for metformin

Correct answer is "d."

Slow-release preparation may be better tolerated in some patients. C Diff infections have closer association with use of antibiotics. Metformin does not cause bowel ischemia. Genetic variations in metformin intolerance exist and this is an area of interest in research.

McCreight, Laura J et al. "Metformin and the gastrointestinal tract." *Diabetologia* vol. 59,3 (2016): 426-35. doi:10.1007/s00125-015-3844-9

Question 8.53

The common nutritional deficiencies seen in obstetric patients after Roux- en-Y gastric bypass surgery include all the following EXCEPT.

a. Vitamin C

b. Iron

c. Folate

d. Vitamin D

e. Vitamin B12

The correct answer is "a."

The common nutritional deficiencies after Roux-en-Y gastric bypass surgery are of protein, iron, vitamin B12, folate, vitamin D, and calcium.
It is important to recognize specific dietary and micronutrient needs of pregnant women who have undergone Roux-en-Y gastric bypass surgery. Vitamin A needs to be in the form of beta-carotene. 5000 IU is the recommended dose. Vitamin A has teratogenic effects. B12 should be given in a dose of 1mg intramuscular every third month. Thiamine recommendations include 50mg daily. Dose may need to be increased in patient with poor intake with excessive nausea or vomiting. Such patients carry risk of developing Wernicke's encephalopathy. Folic acid recommendation is 400 mcg in first 12 weeks and 5mg in later weeks.
Elevated risk of deficiencies demand monitoring of labs in each trimester.

ACOG Practice Bulletin No. 105: Bariatric Surgery and...: Obstetrics & Gynecology. (n.d.). Retrieved January 06, 2018, from http://journals.lww.com/greenjournal/Citation/2009/06000/ACOG_Practice_Bulletin_No__105__Bariatric_Surgery.48.aspx

Question 8.54

A morbidly obese 30-year-old female is referred to her OB/GYN physician for counseling about appropriate birth control options. She is on a combination oral contraceptive pill regimen. She is also following with a bariatric practice. She is using Topiramate phentermine combination for the last couple of months for weight loss. Which of the following statements is correct?

a. The patient may experience breakthrough bleeding
b. Ethinyl estradiol levels may become lower by 30% with concurrent topiramate use
c. Ethinyl estradiol levels may become higher by 30% with concurrent topiramate use
d. Ethinyl estradiol levels are not changed with concurrent topiramate use
e. Norethindrone levels are increased by 50% with concurrent topiramate use
f. a and b are correct

The correct answer is "f."

It has been observed that levels of estrogen component of oral contraceptive pills may become lower with concurrent use of topiramate. This can result in breakthrough bleedings.

Rosenfeld, W. E., Doose, D. R., Walker, S. A., & Nayak, R. K. (1997). Effect of Topiramate on the Pharmacokinetics of an Oral Contraceptive Containing Norethindrone and Ethinyl Estradiol in Patients with Epilepsy. Epilepsia, 38(3), 317-323. doi:10.1111/j.1528-1157.1997.tb01123.x

Question 8.55

Twenty-four y/o female patient gravida 0 presents with complaints of oligomenorrhea, excessive facial hair and weight gain. Physical exam shows BMI 41, hirsutism, acanthosis nigricans, abdominal striae with pannus, and Tanner's stage IV development. Patient's workup shows negative urine pregnancy test, elevated HbA1C, elevated fasting blood sugar, deranged lipid profile, elevated fasting serum insulin, elevated free testosterone, normal DHEAS, normal 17 hydroxyprogesterone acetate, normal TSH and normal prolactin. 24-hour urinary free cortisol excretion test is normal. Which of the following differential diagnoses is suspected?

a. Adrenal hyperplasia

b. PCOS (polycystic ovarian syndrome)

c. Cushing's syndrome

d. Hypothyroidism

e. Hyperprolactinemia

The correct answer is "b."

Question 8.56

What would be the next management steps in the case discussed above?

a. Pelvic ultrasound
b. Progesterone challenge followed by combined birth control pills
c. Metformin
d. Counseling about weight loss and healthy lifestyle
e. All the above statements are correct

The correct answer is "e."

Question 8.57

A 23-year-old female is seeing her family physician for annual physical. She is thinking to start oral contraceptives for birth control. She has concerns about weight gain with the use of this type of contraception. Please select the correct statement.

a. Current oral contraceptives have a great potential to cause weight gain due to estrogen content
b. Fat storage is more likely than fluid retention to cause weight gain with use of oral contraceptives

c. Older contraceptives had high estrogen content, and these were more likely to cause weight gain.
d. Progesterone component of oral contraceptives is a likely factor in causing weight gain

The correct answer is “c.”

Older oral contraceptives which were available several decades ago, had high estrogen levels. These led to weight gain by increasing hunger and fluid retention, in many women. Current generation of oral contraceptives have low estrogens. These are not thought to cause significant weight gain. Any patient using these medications should be aware of these facts. Dietary counseling may help in the patients prone to gain weight.

Question 8.58

Please select the correct statement regarding interaction of naltrexone bupropion (Contrave ®) combination with other medicines.

a. No need of adjusting dose while taking clopidogrel
b. Clopidogrel dose need to be increased while taking naltrexone bupropion combination
c. Clopidogrel interaction with naltrexone/bupropion combination occurs due to inhibition of cytochrome CYP2B6 by the former.
d. Dextromethorphan containing cough suppressant can be used safely with naltrexone/bupropion combination

The correct answer is “c.”

Clopidogrel inhibits cytochrome CYP2B6. This will impair the metabolism of the naltrexone/bupropion combination. This requires the dose of this combination to be reduced. Anti-opioid component "naltrexone" will render opioids ineffective if used concurrently.
https://contravehcp.com/dosing/

Question 8.59

A patient is taking bupropion for reasons of depression. She is not taking any other medications currently. Her BMI is 34. She is interested in trying phentermine to help lose weight. Her family physician discusses the potential risks and benefits of using phentermine and bupropion together. Select the correct statement.

a. Risk of seizures will be increased
b. Two medicines can be used safely. No interaction is expected
c. Risk of arrhythmias increases
d. Dose of phentermine needs to be increased
e. Effect of phentermine will be blunted if used together with bupropion

The correct answer is "a."
Risk of seizures may increase with concurrent use of phentermine and bupropion.
https://www.drugs.com/drug-interactions/phentermine-with-wellbutrin-1851-0-440-203.html#:~:text=buPROPion%20phentermine&text=BuPROPion%20may%20rarely%20cause%20seizures,phentermine%20may%20increase%20that%20risk.

Question 8.60

Phentermine and bupropion combined use risk related to seizures increases in which of the following circumstances?

a. Elderly age group
b. History of brain trauma
c. Alcohol or drug withdrawal
d. Presence of brain tumor
e. All above are correct

The correct answer is "e."
All the choices are correct.
https://www.drugs.com/drug-interactions/phentermine-with-wellbutrin-1851-0-440-203.html#:~:text=buPROPion%20phentermine&text=BuPROPion%20may%20rarely%20cause%20seizures,phentermine%20may%20increase%20that%20risk.

Question 8.61

Which of the following anesthetic has shown to reduce post operative use of narcotics and better pain control in Bariatric patients?

a. Dexmedetomidine (DEX)
b. Nitrous oxide
c. Halothane
d. isoflurane

The correct answer is "a."
Dexmedetomidine belongs to alpha-2 adrenergic receptor agonist family. It produces its beneficial effect probably by reducing the surge of catecholamines and reduced need of volatile anesthetics and opioid agents.

Jin S, Liang DD, Chen C, Zhang M, Wang J. Dexmedetomidine prevent postoperative nausea and vomiting on patients during general anesthesia: A PRISMA-compliant meta-analysis of randomized controlled trials. Medicine (Baltimore). 2017;96(1):e5770. doi:10.1097/MD.0000000000005770

Question 8.62

Thrombotic events after bariatric surgery remain a concerning issue. Better evaluation can help decide about extended DVT prophylaxis. Studies have included panels focusing on factor VIII, protein C, protein S, antithrombin III, and activated protein C resistance. Please select the correct statement

a. Factor VIII elevation is most common anomaly
b. Factor VIII deficiency is most common anomaly
c. Protein C and S deficiency is most common anomaly
d. Protein C resistance is most common anomaly

The correct answer is "a."

Thrombophilia is prevalent in in more than 50% patients seeking sleeve gastrectomy procedure. Factor VIII elevation is found to be the most common anomaly. Extended chemoprophylaxis may decrease portal vein thrombosis risk.
https://link.springer.com/article/10.1007/s11695-009-9906-7

Question 8.63

In bariatric practice a term "carbohydrate loading" is used. Please select the statement which describes this term correctly?

a. It is the bulk of carbohydrate taken before a ketogenic diet protocol is started
b. It is the parenteral carbohydrate load given once nutritional rehabilitation started for a severely malnourished case after any malabsorptive procedure
c. It is the carbohydrate containing drink given on the day of bariatric surgery a couple of hours before anesthesia for various benefits
d. It refers to the carbohydrate load ingested in very low-calorie diet protocols.

The correct answer is "c."

Carbohydrate loading refers to carbohydrate containing drink about 2 hours before the procedure. This helps to reduce insulin resistance, decreases protein loss, and decrease hospital stay. It is shown not affect gastric emptying adversely.

Kratzing C. Pre-operative nutrition and carbohydrate loading. Proc Nutr Soc. 2011 Aug;70(3):311-5. doi: 10.1017/S0029665111000450. PMID: 21781358.

Question 8.64

Thromboembolic complications after bariatric surgery have always been a big concern. Pulmonary embolism is one of the most common causes of mortality after bariatric surgery. Different dosing regimens are used to achieve therapeutic effect with enoxaparin in post operative period. It is estimated that about 15% of morbidly obese patients remain subtherapeutic once given enoxaparin. There are concerns of overdosing as well. Which of the following can be used to determine the adequacy of prophylaxis?

a. Anti-factor Xa
b. Anti-factor XI
c. Anti-factor VII
d. Anti-factor V

The correct answer is "a."
Anti-factor Xa can be used to a assess the adequacy of thromboprophylaxis. It is checked generally 3 to 5 hours after the second dose of enoxaparin.

Assessment of empiric body mass index-based thromboprophylaxis dosing of enoxaparin after bariatric surgery: evidence for dosage adjustment using anti-factor Xa in high-risk patients
Linden A. Karas, M.D. Zubaidah Nor Hanipah, M.D. Derrik Cetin D.O. et al

Question 8.65
A pharmacy service contacts the physician regarding a patient's medication profile. Patient is post gastric sleeve surgery 3 years ago. The note from the pharmacy raises concerns about pantoprazole sodium. Patients insurance claim records also reveal presence of anemia. Please select the correct statement.

a. Iron deficiency could be contributing to the anemia
b. B12 deficiency could be contributing to the anemia
c. PPI related hypochlorhydria can impair the absorption of iron
d. More intensive iron therapy may be necessary
e. All the above statements are correct

The correct answer is "e."

All the statements are correct. Use of PPI can lead to hypochlorhydria leading to iron and B12 malabsorption.

Question 8.66

A patient with sleeve gastrectomy is suffering from severe symptoms of GERD. He is started on Pantoprazole sodium once daily. Symptoms fail to improve. Dose of pantoprazole is adjusted and now he takes BID dose. Symptoms get controlled. Patient stays on this regimen for more than a year. Pharmacy sends a letter to the prescribing physician with concerns regarding high dose of PPI for long duration. Letter mentions some nutritional deficiency risks. High dose and chronic use of pantoprazole may result in deficiency of which of the following

a. Potassium
b. Magnesium
c. sodium
d. zinc
e. All the above statements are correct

The correct answer is "b."

Chronic high dose use of pantoprazole may result in hypomagnesemia.

Question 8.67

Bariatric surgery can affect thyroid status. Which of the following may be expected after significant weight loss?

a. Resolution of subclinical hypothyroidism, decreased TSH level, decreased levothyroxine dose
b. Resolution of subclinical hypothyroidism, increased TSH level, and increased levothyroxine dose
c. No effect on hypothyroidism, TSH level unchanged and decreased dose of levothyroxine
d. Worsening of subclinical hypothyroidism, increased TSH level and no change of levothyroxine dose
e. All the above statements are correct

The correct answer is "a."
A recently published metanalysis determines that bariatric surgery has association with resolution of subclinical hypothyroidism, decreased TSH levels and need of decreased dose of levothyroxine.

Hypothyroidism and levothyroxine therapy following bariatric surgery: a systematic review, meta-analysis, network metanalysis, and meta- regression CArmil Azran,Pham.D., Nirvana Hanhan-Shamshoum, Tujan Irshied Soard Voume 17, Issue 6 P1206-1217

Question 8.68

Clinical practice guidelines recommend

a. Avoid using extended-release ER formulations in post bariatric surgery situations
b. Absorption surface area is increased for extended-release formulations in a gastric bypass patient due to rerouting of bowel
c. Intermediate-release (IR) and non-absorbable sugar containing liquid formulations are not preferred in post bariatric surgery patients.
d. Efficacy of extended-release medications is increased after gastric bypass surgery
e. All the above statements are correct

The correct answer is "a."
Based upon a recent study it appears that extended-release preparations should be avoided in post bariatric patients. This study looked at the data related gastric bypass and sleeve gastrectomy patients. Potential untoward effects are attributed to the use of extended-release formulations in this category of the patients.
Changes in utilization of immediate-release, extended-release, and liquid formulation medications relative to bariatric surgery: a segmented regression analysis Scott Martin Vouri 1, Hemita Bhagwandass 2, et all Obes Relat Dis. Surg 2021 Jun;17(6):1089-1094. doi: 10.1016/j.soard.2021.02.027. Epub 2021 Mar 3.

Question 8.69

Morbidly obese patients are vulnerable to have thiamine deficiency. Please select the correct statement.

a. Females with shorter height are likely to have higher thiamine levels
b. Taller males are likely to have higher thiamine levels
c. Human body have stores of thiamine which can be sufficient for many months
d. Adipose tissues are rich in thiamine
e. All the above statements are correct

The correct answer is "b."

Human body has limited thiamine stores. Skeletal muscles have higher concentration of thiamine. Taller males with more muscular mass are likely to have higher thiamine levels. Obese patients in perioperative period are more vulnerable to thiamine deficiency. This can have serious neurological consequences including Korsakoff psychosis or Wernicke encephalopathy.

Prevalence of thiamine deficiency is significant in patients undergoing primary bariatric surgery

VAncel. Albaugh, M.D., Brandon Williams, M.D. et all

Question 8.70

Vitamin E plays role in several body processes. Please select the correct statement.

a. Vitamin E is a fat-soluble vitamin
b. Vitamin E deficiency is some time seen in post bariatric surgery patients
c. Patients with malabsorption type bariatric procedures are affected more
d. Vitamin E is stored predominantly in adipose tissues
e. Neuropathy, myopathy, gait disturbances, sensory loss, ataxia, immune disorders, and ophthalmologic deficits are some of the clinical manifestations of the deficiency
f. All the above are correct

The correct answer is "f."
Vitamin E is a one of the fat-soluble vitamins. It is found in plants. Seeds, nuts, green leafy vegetables, vegetable oils and fish naturally contain this vitamin. In human body its benefits include antioxidant properties, immune effects, modulation of enzymes and signal transduction. This vitamin is mainly absorbed in proximal bowel. Dose recommendations are not well defined at present.
Vitamin E status among bariatric surgery patients: a systematic review
Shiri Sherf-Degn, R.D., PhD, Assaf Buch R.D., Ph.D, et all

Question 8.71

Please select the correct statement regarding use of vitamins in pregnant patients

a. Retinoids are not safe to use during pregnancy
b. Beta carotenes can be used in pregnancy
c. B12 and folic acid are teratogenic
d. Options "a." and "b." are correct
e. All the above statements are correct

The correct answer is "d."

Question 8.72

Dexmedetomidine has been in focus in Bariatric surgery. What is the pharmacological importance of this medication?

a. It is a betablocker. It helps control heart rate
b. It is a highly selective alpha-2 adrenergic receptor agonist. It is found useful in post operative nausea control
c. It is a weight loss medication
d. It helps control Binge eating

The correct answer is "b."

Question 8.73

Select the correct statement regarding Dexmedetomidine therapeutic effects.

a. Sedation
b. Analgesia
c. Anxiolytic
d. Less respiratory depression
e. All above statements are correct

The correct answer is “e.”
Dexmedetomidine has gained interest regarding prevention of postoperative nausea after bariatric surgery. A lot of emphasis is being made recently to cut down use of narcotics in bariatric surgery practice. ”BStop” initiative is one the quality improvement projects by the leading organizations in the field. This medicine is found beneficial regarding reducing the dose of opioids in the perioperative period. It is also shown to cause appreciable reduction in postoperative pain scores.
Editorial Comment on: Postoperative nausea and vomiting after bariatric surgery and dexmedetomidine anesthetic: a propensity-weighted analysis. Surgery for Obesity and Related Disease 16 (2020) e39-e40

Question 8.74

Iron absorption can be altered in certain situations. Please select the correct statement regarding oral iron therapy.

a. Absorption of iron can be impaired if calcium and iron are taken at the same time
b. Absorption of iron is enhanced if it is taken along with calcium
c. Absorption of iron is decreased if vitamin C is taken concurrently
d. All the above statements are correct

The correct answer is "a."
Iron absorption can be impaired if it is taken along with calcium. Timing of intake of calcium and iron should be at least 2 hours apart. Low calcium content is seen in some dedicated bariatric vitamin preparations for the same reasons.

Question 8.75

Please select the correct statement about use of specialized vitamins after bariatric surgery.

a. It is not important to take specialized vitamins after bariatric surgery
b. Taking specialized vitamins is more important in prevention of various deficiencies in sleeve gastrectomy patients only.
c. Taking specialized vitamins is more important in prevention of various deficiencies in gastric bypass patients
d. Taking specialized vitamins is more important in prevention of various deficiencies in gastric adjustable band patients.

The correct answer is "c."
Gastric bypass patient may see deficiencies more often related to iron, B12, folic acid, and vitamin D. Malabsorption and small stomach size contributes various nutritional deficiencies.
Do specialized bariatric multivitamins lower deficiencies after RYGB
Wendy Schijns, MD, Lisanne T. Schuurman, MD, Alida Melse-Boonstra, MD et al Surgery for Obesity and Related Disease 14(2018) 1005-1002

Question 8.76

Warfarin management in perioperative period in bariatric patients poses several challenges. Please select the correct statement.

a. Warfarin is mainly absorbed in terminal ileum, so its dose and levels are not affected by a Roux-en-Y gastric bypass.
b. It is observed that in gastric bypass patients dose requirements tend to be lower in first month and later increase
c. Warfarin is mainly metabolized in renal tissues
d. Warfarin dose requires to be increased in immediate post operative period as most absorption of warfarin occurs in proximal duodenum.

The correct answer is "b."
Warfarin is mainly absorbed in proximal duodenum however due to various other factors not completely understood, the dose requirements remain lower in immediate postoperative period after gastric bypass. A dose reduction by approximately 25% or more may be required in early post operative period. Warfarin is metabolized in liver by enzymes CYP2C9 and CYP3A4 of cytochrome p450 group.

Andew T. Strong, MD, Guatam Sharma et al SOARD VOLUME 14 ISSUE 5 P700-706 MAY 01 2018

https://doi.org/10.1016/j.soard.2017.12021

Question 8.77

Which of the following medications have shown some benefit in Obese patients with diabetes and non-alcoholic fatty liver disease?

a. Metformin.
b. Liraglutide
c. Sitagliptin
d. Pioglitazone

The correct answer is "d."
Pioglitazone has shown some improvement in numbers regarding haptic fat content. No improvement is noted in fibrosis scores. Patient on pioglitazone can have some weight gain.

Blazina, I., Selph, S. Diabetes drugs for nonalcoholic fatty liver disease: a systematic review. Syst Rev 8, 295 (2019). https://doi.org/10.1186/s13643-019-1200-8

Question 8.78

A patient who is following a weight loss program calls to have an appointment to discuss trying semaglutide. She read about this medicine on internet. Please select the correct statement.

a. This a GLP1 agonist
b. It is once a week injectable preparation for weight loss.
c. It cannot be used in patients with history of medullary thyroid cancer or Type 2 multiple endocrine neoplasia syndrome
d. Some of the side effects include, pancreatitis, gallstones, renal impairment, risk of hypoglycemia, depression, and suicidal ideations

e. All the above statements are correct

correct answer is "e."
Semaglutide (Wegovy ™) * is a glucagon-like peptide-1 (GLP-1) agonist. This injectable medication increases secretion of insulin. It is given once a week and dose is titrated to a higher level with monthly increments. An oral version of this medicine is available to treat diabetes.

https://en.wikipedia.org/wiki/Semaglutide#cite_note-FDA2019-18
https://www.wegovy.com/?gclid=Cj0KCQjwnoqLBhD4ARIsAL5JedJCUJgSctJNitfXT2Tljmaxq7J_oeZ65M-YUZE1pxjPDgUUmSuWDQEaArVQEALw_wcB&gclsrc=aw.ds
* Wegovy™ is a trademark of Novo Nordisk A/S.

Question 8.79

Please select the correct statement about semaglutide?

a. Dose adjustment is needed in patients with renal impairment
b. Dose adjustment is needed in patients with hepatic impairment
c. Dose adjustment is needed in patients with both renal and hepatic impairments
d. Dose adjustment is not needed in patients with both renal and hepatic impairments

The correct answer is "d."
Semaglutide (Wegovy ™) clinical trial has shown no clinically relevant change in patients with both renal and hepatic impairments. However, it should be kept in mind that symptoms related to nausea, vomiting and diarrhea can lead to acute renal injury especially in patients with preexisting renal impairment. In clinical trials it has been used in patients

above 65 years of age. Safety and efficacy were comparable to younger patients
https://www.novo-pi.com/wegovy.pdf

Question 8.80

Semaglutide should be discontinued before planned pregnancy. It is suggested that the drug should be discontinued at least how much time before?

a. 5 days
b. 10 days
c. 2 weeks
d. 4 weeks
e. 2 months

The correct answer is "e."
Semaglutide has a long half-life of 1 week. Drug may be present in the body system 4 to 7 weeks following a dose of 2.4 mg. Extensive binding to plasma protein slows its degradation and clearance through the kidneys.
https://www.novo-pi.com/wegovy.pdf

Question 8.81

Please select the correct statement about Semaglutide

a. Its action through GLP 1 receptors include reduction of insulin production
b. Its action through GLP 1 receptors include increased production of insulin
c. Its action through GLP 1 receptors include reduction of glucagon production
d. Its action through GLP 1 receptors include increased production of glucagon
e. Options (b) and (c) are correct

The correct answer is "e."
Semaglutide (Wegovy ™) causes increased production of insulin and decreases production of glucagon. These effects help in lowering blood sugar.
https://www.novo-pi.com/wegovy.pdf

Question 8.82

Semaglutide is GLP1 analogue, and it acts through GLP 1 receptors

a. Semaglutide acts through its action on GLP 1 receptors present in pancreas
b. Semaglutide acts through its action on GLP 1 receptors present in Liver
c. Semaglutide acts through its action on GLP 1 receptors present in fat cells
d. Semaglutide acts through its action on GLP 1 receptors present in brain
e. Options (a) and (b) are correct

The correct answer is "d."
Semaglutide acts through its action on appetite control centers in brain by its action on GLP1 receptors.
https://www.novo-pi.com/wegovy.pdf

Question 8.83

Please select the correct statement about ICG (indocyanine green dye) use in management of obese patients

a. Can be used to assess fatty liver
b. Can help visualize biliary ductal structures during bariatric surgery and concurrent cholecystectomy
c. Can help assess vascularity of tissues during bariatric surgical procedures
d. Can help assess anastomosis integrity by injecting in the stomach
e. All the above statements are correct

The correct answer is "e."
ICG dye is used very commonly in surgical practices. It produces fluorescent green color. This can be picked with special cameras during laparoscopic / robotic and other procedures. This property makes it useful to identify vascularity of tissues in addition to the uses mentioned above.
Carrano, F. M., & Di Lorenzo, N. (2020). The use of indocyanine green in bariatric surgery: A systematic review. Journal of Gastric Surgery, 2(2), 41–44. https://doi.org/10.36159/jgs.v2i2.47

Question 8.84

Which of the following chemotherapeutic agents should be given according to predicted normal weight of an obese patient?

a. Paclitaxel
b. Troxacitabine
c. Irinotecan
d. Cicplatin
e. Carboplatin

The correct answer is "e."
Doses of options (a) to (d) should be calculated according to surface area. However, carboplatin should be dosed according to predicted normal weight of the patient.
https://journals.lww.com/oncology-times/fulltext/2012/02250/how_obesity_complicates_cancer_treatment.1.aspx

Question 8.85

Tendencies among oncologists exist to reduce the doses of various chemotherapeutic agents to lessen risks of toxicity in obese patients. Please select the correct statement about American society of clinical oncology guidelines regarding dosing issue.

a. Panel suggest full weight-based dosing of cytotoxic chemotherapeutic agents
b. Full approved doses of immune and targeted therapies in obese adults cancer patients
c. In case of toxicity doses should be modified and handled similarly in nonobese and obese patients

d. Fixed dose therapy is limited to select cytotoxic agents like bleomycin
e. All above statements are correct

The correct answer is "e."
Guidelines published in 2021 state the above facts.
DOI: 10.1200/JCO.21.00471 Journal of Clinical Oncology 39, no. 18 (June 20, 2021) 2037-2048.

Question 8.86

There is limited data about dosing guidelines for many commonly used medications in critically sick obese patients. Which of the following medications is recommended to have standard dose without size descriptor?

a. Non opioid analgesics
b. ketamine
c. Opioid analgesics
d. None of the above medications is recommended to have dosing without size descriptor

The correct answer is "a."
Non opioids are recommended to be used with standard doses. For Ketamine and opioids, ideal or adjusted body weight should be used to calculate doses.
Erstad, B.L., Barletta, J.F. Drug dosing in the critically ill obese patient—a focus on sedation, analgesia, and delirium. Crit Care 24, 315 (2020). https://doi.org/10.1186/s13054-020-03040-z

Question 8.87

Which of the following sedative medications are recommended to be used according to actual body weight when BMI is less than 40 kg/m^2 ?

a. Propofol
b. Midazolam
c. Dexmedetomidine
d. Etomidate

The correct answer is "d."
Etomidate is recommended to be used with actual body weight when BMI is less than 40 and for BMI more than 40 adjusted or actual body weight should be used. For propofol, Dexmedetomidine and Midazolam ideal or adjusted body weight should be used. Similarly ideal weight should be used for midazolam while giving infusions.
Erstad, B.L., Barletta, J.F. Drug dosing in the critically ill obese patient—a focus on sedation, analgesia, and delirium. Crit Care 24, 315 (2020). https://doi.org/10.1186/s13054-020-03040-z

Question 8.88

Which of the following medications can be used with standard, non-weight-based doses in obese critically sick patients?

a. Propofol
b. Quetiapine
c. Dexmedetomidine
d. Haloperidol
e. Options (b) and (d) are correct

The correct answer is "d."
Quetiapine and haloperidol are used with standard, non-weigh-based doses.
Erstad, B.L., Barletta, J.F. Drug dosing in the critically ill obese patient—a focus on sedation, analgesia, and delirium. Crit Care 24, 315 (2020). https://doi.org/10.1186/s13054-020-03040-z

Question 8.89

A 55-year-old female who is post Roux-en-Y gastric bypass develops internal hernia with strangulation. Major small bowel resection was done. After a long hospital stay, she is discharged to a rehab facility with total parenteral nutritional support. She is counseled about her future options to manage short bowel syndrome. Which of the following medications can potentially help her?

a. GLP-1 agonist
b. Leptin injections
c. GLP-2 agonist
d. Insulin injections

Correct answer is "c."

Teduglutide (brand name Gattex) is a GLP-2 agonist. It promotes mucosal growth, gastric emptying, and stomach secretions. Development of tumors, hepatobiliary disease, fluid overload, intestinal obstruction and altered absorption of some of the drugs are few of the side effects. Potential for various malignancies is a concerning issue. Leptin and insulin have no specific role in short bowel syndrome management. GLP 1 agonists have been used in treatment of diabetes and lately also for weight loss.

Physiology of Weight Maintenance

Question 9.1

A morbidly obese patient has been treated in a bariatric practice. He lost significant weight. He is interested in finding out how he can maintain weight for years to come. Which of the following levels measured during weight loss may be useful in predicting the future outcome?

a. Fasting Insulin level
b. HbA1c level
c. TSH level
d. Angiotensin-converting enzyme level
e. None of the above are useful in predicting future weight loss.

The correct answer is "d."

A study by Wang et al. concluded that a reduction in the level of the angiotensin-converting enzyme might be a useful tool to predict long-term weight loss.

Wang, P., Holst, C., Wodzig, W. K., Andersen, M. R., Astrup, A., Baak, M. A., . . . Mariman, E. C. (2012). Circulating ACE is a predictor of weight loss maintenance not only in overweight and obese women but also in men. International Journal of Obesity, 36(12), 1545-1551. doi:10.1038/ijo.2011.278

Question 9.2

American College of Sports Medicine published guidelines to address the amount and type of activity to maintain a healthy weight. Please select the correct statement.

a. 30 to 45 minutes of moderate-intensity activity per week is likely to prevent weight gain

b. 50 to 75 minutes of moderate-intensity activity per week is expected to prevent weight gain

c. 100 to 125 minutes of moderate-intensity activity per week is likely to prevent weight gain

d. 130 to 150 minutes of moderate-intensity activity per week is expected to prevent weight gain

e. 200 to 300 minutes of moderate-intensity activity per week is likely to prevent weight gain

The correct answer is "e."

Activity with moderate intensity for a duration up to 5 hours a week is generally needed to maintain weight.

Donnelly, J. E., Blair, S. N., Jakicic, J. M., Manore, M. M., Rankin, J. W., & Smith, B. K. (2009). Appropriate Physical Activity Intervention Strategies for Weight Loss and Prevention of Weight Regain for Adults. Medicine & Science in Sports & Exercise, 41(2), 459-471. doi:10.1249/mss.0b013e3181949333

Question 9.3

In recent years, there has been interest in exploring the relationship of gut microbiome with obesity. Which of the following statements is correct?

a. Firmicutes predominance is associated with obesity
b. Firmicutes predominance is associated with leaner weight
c. Bacteroidetes predominance is associated with obesity
d. Bacteroidetes predominance is associated with more energy harvesting
e. Firmicutes predominance is associated with less energy harvesting

The correct answer is "a."

There is interest in recent years about the role of gut microbiota in energy balance. It has been shown that Bacteroidetes predominance is associated with relatively leaner weight.

Brestoff, J. R., & Artis, D. (2013). Commensal bacteria at the interface of host metabolism and the immune system. Nature Immunology, 14(7), 676-684. doi:10.1038/ni.2640

Question 9.4

The term (MHO) stands for “Metabolically Healthy but Obese” individuals. Which of the following statements is correct about this condition?

a. MHO individuals are at less risk to develop metabolic syndrome
b. MHO individuals are at increased risk of cardiac disease and failure
c. MHO individuals are at low risk of cardiac disease and failure
d. Sleep apnea and cancer risk is low in individuals with HMO
e. None of the above statements is true.

The correct answer is "b."

Increased risk of cardiac disease and cardiac failure exists in people with MHO.

“Nonalcoholic Steatohepatitis (NASH).” PathologyBays, H E. “Adiposopathy Is ‘Sick Fat’ a cardiovascular disease?” Current Neurology and Neuroscience Reports., U.S. National Library of Medicine, 21 June 2011, www.ncbi.nlm.nih.gov/pubmed/21679848.Outlines - PathologyOutlines.com, www.pathologyoutlines.com/topic/liverNASH.html.

Issues Related to Bariatric Surgery Patients

Question 10.1

A 35-year-old female with BMI of 43 is interested in bariatric surgery option for weight loss. A screening lab panel is done. Vitamin D level is found low. Which of the following statements is correct?

a. Vitamin D deficiency is seen in up to two-thirds of cases seeking bariatric surgical options
b. Her parathyroid hormone level is likely to be low
c. Vitamin D deficiency is most likely due to an absorption defect
d. Screening test for vitamin D is a cost-effective test, and it should be used liberally for screening and follow up
e. Over the counter multivitamins generally contain enough vitamin D to help replenish the deficiency

The correct answer is "a."

Bioavailability of vitamin D is one of the factors leading to low vitamin D in obese patients. Parathyroid level tends to be somewhat raised. Testing for vitamin D is generally not cost effective. Higher doses of vitamin D are needed to replenish the deficiency.

Kaidar-Person, O., & Rosenthal, R. J. (2007). Commentary Regarding Flancbaum L, Belsley S, Drake V, Colarusso T, Tayler E. Preoperative Nutritional Status of Patients Undergoing

Roux-en-Y Gastric Bypass for Morbid Obesity. J Gastrointest Surg. 2006 10(7):1033–7. Journal of Gastrointestinal Surgery, 12(2), 397-397. doi:10.1007/s11605-007-0429-z

Question 10.2

Which of the following deficiencies is seen most commonly in morbidly obese patients?

a. Iron
b. Folic acid
c. B12
d. Vitamin D
e. B1

The correct answer is "d."

Vitamin D deficiency remains one of the most common deficiencies in a population suffering from obesity.

Kaidar-Person, O., & Rosenthal, R. J. (2007). Commentary Regarding Flancbaum L, Belsley S, Drake V, Colarusso T, Tayler E. Preoperative Nutritional Status of Patients Undergoing Roux-en-Y Gastric Bypass for Morbid Obesity. J Gastrointest Surg. 2006 10(7):1033–7. Journal of Gastrointestinal Surgery, 12(2), 397-397. doi:10.1007/s11605-007-0429-z

Question 10.3

A patient had Biliopancreatic diversion operation for weight loss eight years ago. She did not have regular follow up with her bariatric center. Currently, she does not take any dietary or vitamin supplements. She has started experiencing visual problems for the last few months. Her symptoms are getting progressively worse. It is becoming harder for her to see at night and eyes remain dry. Which of the following vitamin deficiency is expected?

a. Vitamin D

b. Vitamin A

c. Vitamin C

d. Vitamin B6

e. Vitamin B1

The correct answer is "b."

Vitamin A is a fat-soluble vitamin. Patients who undergo biliopancreatic diversion, are more vulnerable (above 50% cases in some reported series). It may also occur in other bariatric procedures like gastric bypass which also has a malabsorptive component.

Question 10.4

A 40 -year-old female with morbid obesity underwent a sleeve gastrectomy procedure for weight loss. Her Bariatric surgeon forwards the discharge summary to her family physician with operative note comments that he observed nodularity of the liver during the procedure. A liver biopsy at the time sleeve gastrectomy was performed. Her pathology report would be available in a few days. She does not have a previous history of hepatitis or alcohol abuse. Her pre-operative EGD did not show any esophageal varices. Which of the following statements is correct?

a. In obese patients, the prevalence of NASH (Nonalcoholic steatohepatitis) is up to 10 %
b. Most obese patients are diagnosed with the presence of cirrhosis of the liver during preoperative workup
c. The surgeon should not have done sleeve gastrectomy in this patient after observing nodularity of the liver
d. She is likely to have more complications during next one year follow up as compared to a person undergoing similar surgery and not having cirrhosis findings
e. NASH is expected to be to be the etiology.

The correct answer is "e."

Question 10.5

Presume the patient discussed in above question was found to have some abnormality of liver functions including mildly raised ALT and AST levels before surgery. She is requested to have a clearance letter for Bariatric Surgery from her PCP. Her family physician requests additional investigations. Which of the following statements is true?

a. An ultrasound done as part of preoperative workup could have likely picked her condition of cirrhosis

b. A liver biopsy is not recommended at the time of surgery

c. Presence of portal hypertension is not considered as a contraindication for bariatric surgery

d. She is likely to have similar weight loss by one year as compared to if she had no cirrhosis

e. NASH is unlikely to improve after bariatric surgery

The correct answer is "d."

NASH is estimated to affect up to 70% of obese patients. This condition may be present in up to 20 percent of the general population. The first clue of the problem comes at the time of surgery when operating surgeon observes the abnormal appearance of the liver. The surgeon can proceed for operation if portal hypertension is not present. Enlarged veins at the hiatus and falciform ligament are suggestive of the presence of portal hypertension. Subsequent follow-up does not show higher complications than patients undergoing surgery who do not have cirrhosis. NASH may improve after weight loss. Similar weight loss is seen in a patient with cirrhosis and without cirrhosis. Liver biopsy done at the time of surgery can give tissue diagnosis with the determination of histological type.

Rebibo, L., Gerin, O., Verhaeghe, P., Dhahri, A., Cosse, C., & Regimbeau, J. (2014). Laparoscopic sleeve gastrectomy in patients with NASH-related cirrhosis: A case-matched study. Surgery for Obesity and Related Diseases, 10(3), 405-410. doi: 10.1016/j.soard.2013.09.015

Question 10.6

A 43-year female had adjustable gastric band surgery ten years ago. She has a history of DM 2 and HTN. Her pre-operative BMI was 39. She lost 40 pounds after surgery, and her current BMI is 33. Which of the following statements is correct about gastric adjustable bands?

a. Gastric adjustable band is currently one of the most commonly done bariatric procedures

b. Most patient receiving adjustable gastric bands have complete resolution of DM at ten years follow up

c. She is unlikely to be using PPI

d. Less than 5% of the patient with gastric adjustable bands will need revisional bariatric procedures by ten years for reasons of complications related to the band itself

e. She is likely to have a low BAROS Score (Bariatric Analysis and Reporting Outcome Scale)

The correct answer is "e."

BAROS Score (Bariatric Analysis and Reporting Outcome Scale) is a scoring system to access quality of life. Scoring with this system looks at weight loss, complications, and reinterventions. Additionally, mental status, physical activity, social issues, work, sexual function, and relation with food are integrated into the score calculations. Patients are grouped into 5 categories form failure to excellent based on the scores obtained. The score itself ranges from negative to a maximum of 9 points.

Aarts, E., Dogan, K., Koehestanie, P., Aufenacker, T., Janssen, I., & Berends, F. (2014). Long-term results after laparoscopic adjustable gastric banding: a mean fourteen-year follow-up study. Surgery for Obesity and Related Diseases, 10(4), 633-640. doi: 10.1016/j.soard.2014.03.019

Question 10.7

A 55-year patient visits his family doctor's office for a pre-bariatric surgery clearance examination. Patient's current BMI is 45. Patient has sleep apnea, hypertension, and uncontrolled diabetes. The patient is currently on insulin and additionally takes metformin. Current A1C is 11. The patient is opting for a Roux-en-Y Gastric Bypass procedure for weight loss and diabetes control. Which of the following statements is correct about A1C and post-bariatric surgery risks?

a. The raised A1C level is associated with increased risks of postoperative complications and high 30 days hospital re-admission rates.

b. The raised A1C level is associated with similar risks of post-operative complications and the same 30 days hospital re-admission rates as with patients with normal A1C levels

c. This patient is more likely to be a female rather than a male

d. Patient with HbA1C levels between 5.7 to 6.6 should always be managed with anti-diabetic medications in pre-operative periods

e. Bariatric surgery should never be offered to patients with increased A1C levels because of risks of complications.

The correct answer is "a."

Elevated levels of A1c without appropriate treatment are associated with adverse outcomes. High 30 days morbidity numbers reflect this.

Surgery for Obesity and Related Disease. 2014; 10:801-807

Question 10.8

A 30-year-old woman had Roux-en-Y gastric bypass five days ago. The patient was discharged on the postoperative day three, in a stable condition. Patient calls her doctor's office. She is complaining of severe left upper abdominal pain with nausea. She describes a temperature of 38° C and a heart rate of 115 per minute.

Which of the following statements is true regarding her clinical condition?

a. She should take an extra dose of acetaminophen hydrocodone
b. Her symptoms are likely due to atelectasis and developing pneumonia
c. Such symptoms are common in most patients after bariatric surgeries
d. She should stop her oral intake and see her family doctor at the earliest available appointment in the coming days.
e. She may be developing an anastomotic leak, and she should be seen in the emergency room as soon as possible to get evaluated.

The correct answer is "e."

This patient presents with features suggestive of anastomotic leak and peritonitis. Patient with tachycardia, distress, and pain symptoms need prompt evaluation. Work up includes clinical examination, white blood counts and imaging studies like CT scan to rule out any anastomotic leak. If a leak is suspected, some invasive intervention is generally needed.

Question 10.9

Which of the following procedures is associated with the highest incidence of malabsorption?

a. Adjustable gastric band
b. Sleeve gastrectomy
c. Roux-en-Y gastric bypass
d. Biliopancreatic Diversion
e. Vertical Banded Gastroplasty

The correct answer is "d."

Biliopancreatic diversion operation is associated with most weight loss. At the same time, this procedure is associated with significant malabsorption, reflected by the high incidence of diarrhea and nutritional deficiencies.

Question 10.10

A 44-year-old patient with 66 BMI undergoes gastric bypass surgery. On postoperative day 2, he complains of shortness of breath. His oxygen saturation is 88% with 8 liters of O2 given through nasal cannula. Which of the following statement is correct about his clinical condition?

a. A CT angiogram of the chest is needed to evaluate his condition further

b. Continue observation. CT scan study should not be done due to radiation risk

c. Inferior vena cava filter should be placed

d. The patient should be immediately taken to operating room to explore the abdomen

e. Antibiotics should be immediately started to treat pneumonia

The correct answer is "a."

Inpatient with super morbid obesity who develop shortness of breath with chest pain and require higher oxygen to maintain should be investigated for pulmonary embolism.

Question 10.11

A 37-year-old patient had adjustable gastric band several years ago. She lost about 40 lbs. She has difficulty in tolerating diet with nausea and vomiting for the last few days. Which of the following statements is <u>not</u> correct regarding her clinical condition and management plan?

a. Emptying of the band should be considered early

b. Upper GI contrast study may be helpful in the evaluation

c. Slippage of the band is one of the differential diagnoses

d. She may need hospital admission for rehydration

e. Gastroesophageal reflux disease is rare in patients receiving adjustable gastric bands

The correct answer is "e."

Pouch dilatation with dilatation of the esophagus with motility problems can be troublesome for most patients. Gastroesophageal reflux-related symptoms are also common. Patients may need emptying of the band and PPIs. A slipped band may require deflation. If symptoms do not improve, she may need operative removal of the gastric band.

Question 10.12

A 46-year-old patient is seen in the emergency room. She had Roux-en-Y gastric several years ago and lost about 90 lbs. She smokes one pack of cigarettes daily and recently experienced increasing difficulty in tolerating diet. She has frequent nausea and vomiting for the last several days. Which of the following statements is correct regarding her clinical condition and management?

a. Upper GI contrast studies are not helpful in such scenarios

b. Vitamin B1 is not needed

c. Gastrojejunal anastomosis stricture should be considered in the differential diagnosis

d. Marginal gastro-jejunal ulcers are unlikely to lead to obstruction at gastro-jejunostomy anastomosis site

e. Esophagogastrojejunoscopy should be used more liberally to see for any marginal ulcers

f. Options “c” and “e” are correct

The correct answer is "f."

Gastrojejunostomy is a delicate balance. Several factors play in the development of local ulcer disease. Patients taking NSAIDs and smokers are more vulnerable. Local ischemia due to loss of blood supply adds to poor healing. Local foreign bodies like sutures and protruding staples should be looked at the endoscopic examination. Gastric fistulae and larger gastric pouch size can contribute to more acid exposure of vulnerable jejunum at the anastomosis to develop marginal ulcers which sometimes lead to stenosis at the anastomosis. Frequent vomiting may cause B1 (thiamine) deficiency. Recognizing this deficiency in such clinical situations is important. Prompt replacement of B1 may prevent some of the undesirable neurological consequences.

Question 10.13

A bariatric surgical procedure will be considered as having <u>insufficient</u> weight loss if

a. If weight loss is 70 to 80 percent of excess weight

b. If weight loss is 60 to 70 percent of excess weight

c. If weight loss is less than 40 to 50% of excess weight

d. If weight loss is more than 50 to 60 % of excess weight

e. Resolution of comorbidities like hypertension and diabetes is not seen

The correct answer is "c."

In general, excess weight loss of less than 40 to 50 percent is considered insufficient after bariatric surgery. However, even this much weight loss still has some significant metabolic benefits.

Question 10.14

All the following are contraindications for Bariatric Surgery <u>Except</u>

a. A female patient who is planning for pregnancy within a year
b. A person currently with active substance abuse.
c. A patient who has suicidal ideations
d. A diabetic patient with HbA1c of 7.5
e. A person with uncontrolled depression

The correct answer is "d."

High A1c levels are associated with high postoperative complication rates. Aggressive treatment of diabetes to bring high A1c levels under control can potentially prevent some the complications in the perioperative period. This fact is supported by several studies in different disciplines including bariatrics and colorectal surgery. It is noted that patients with A1C of higher than 8 have a longer length of stay in the hospital after noncardiac surgery.

Underwood, P., Askari, R., Hurwitz, S., Chamarthi, B., & Garg, R. (2014). Response to Comment on Underwood et al. Preoperative A1C and Clinical Outcomes in Patients With Diabetes Undergoing Major Noncardiac Surgical Procedures. Diabetes Care 2014;37:611–616. Diabetes Care, 37(8). doi:10.2337/dc14-0738

Question 10.15

Which of the following statements is correct regarding the psychology evaluation of patients seeking bariatric surgery?

a. Approximately 25% of patients who seek bariatric surgery may have a diagnosis of an Axis 1 or 2 disorder
b. Mood disorders are the least common disorders seen in Bariatric Surgical candidates
c. Binge eating disorder is a contraindication for bariatric surgery
d. Historically 40 to 50 % of patients are excluded from bariatric surgery based on their psychology evaluation
e. Night eating syndrome is seen in less than 10 % of patients seeking bariatric surgery

The correct answer is "a."

Question 10.16

A patient had Roux-en-Y Gastric bypass seven years ago. He has lost significant weight, and current BMI is 31. He has started smoking for the last six months. He experienced pain in the epigastric area and had frequent nausea. He vomits food very often. All the following statements are correct about his management except

a. Upper GI contrast study may help in the evaluation.
b. Upper GI endoscopy will be needed in most cases of similar symptoms
c. Marginal ulcer and stenosis of gastrojejunostomy is a likely diagnosis
d. Patients with similar symptoms can also have a B1 deficiency
e. Laparoscopic or open revision of gastrojejunostomy should be planned urgently as the approach of endoscopic dilatations frequently fails.

The correct answer is "e."

Counseling to stop smoking should be done with the provision of resources to help quit this habit. Options including upper GI endoscopy and contrast study can be used for evaluation. Marginal ulcer and its sequelae of stenosis at gastrojejunostomy can explain the symptoms of pain, nausea, and vomiting. Medical measures including proton pump inhibitors along with cytoprotective medications should be considered. Patients need to improve their protein intake. Most cases of stenosis at anastomosis respond to dilatation. In the presence of smoking any revisional surgery attempt is likely to be unsuccessful.

Question 10.17

A patient who had Roux-en-Y Gastric bypass surgery in the past presents with upper
GI symptoms. She feels nausea, palpitations, dizziness, flushing, diarrhea, and syncopal symptoms after meals. Dumping syndrome is expected. Which of the following statements is correct about her clinical condition?

a. Her symptoms are more likely to be due to the intake of proteins.

b. Dumping syndrome symptoms tend to continue for many years in most patients.

c. Symptoms tend to improve with large infrequent meals

d. Bradycardia and decreased level of glucagon-like peptide (GLP-1) are expected

e. Tachycardia and increased level of glucagon-like peptide (GLP-1) is expected

The correct answer is "e."

Classically dumping symptom occurs in first six months after gastric bypass surgery. Patients experience symptoms of pain in abdomen, vomiting, nausea, flushing, diarrhea, dizziness, weakness, headaches, and increased heart rate after taking high sugar diets. Most cases resolve spontaneously over time. Patients are encouraged to make dietary modifications. Small frequent meals usually help. Several mechanisms may be contributing to this disorder. High glucagon-like peptide and beta cell hyperplasia are suspected underlying etiologies.

Abell, T. L., & Minocha, A. (2006). Gastrointestinal Complications of Bariatric Surgery: Diagnosis and Therapy. The American Journal of the Medical Sciences, 331(4), 214-218. doi:10.1097/00000441-200604000-00008

Question 10.18

The resolution of diabetes is more likely to be observed in which of the following procedures?

a. Adjustable gastric band
b. Vertical banded gastroplasty
c. Roux-en-Y Gastric Bypass
d. Sleeve Gastrectomy
e. Intra-gastric balloon

The correct answer is "c."

Out of all the above-listed procedures, Roux-en-Y gastric bypass has best results as far as control of diabetes is concerned. Lowering of blood sugar is seen very shortly after gastric bypass even before any significant weight loss is observed. Type 2 diabetes improves in 90 % of cases and in up to 78% of cases it goes into remission.
STAMPEDE clinical trial shows patients with type 2 diabetes undergoing bariatric surgery with intense medical therapy do

better than patients treated with intense medical therapy alone. A1c improves more in patients receiving Roux-en-Y gastric bypass.

Surgery for Diabetes – ASMBS Learning Center. (n.d.). Retrieved December 29, 2017, from https://asmbs.org/patients/surgery-for-diabetes

Question 10.19

A 42-year-old morbidly obese female with type 2 DM is seeking advice for bariatric surgery. She has a BMI of 45 and weighs 265 lbs. She sees her family physician for pre-surgery clearance. She is concerned about her diabetes. She asks questions about the chances of remission of her DM after the bariatric procedure. Which of the following can better predict post-surgery remission of diabetes?

a. C Peptide is a better predictor of post-op remission of diabetes
b. C- Peptide AUC (area under the curve after glucose tolerance test) is a better predictor of post-op remission of diabetes
c. HbA1C level
d. Age of the patient
e. Duration of Diabetes

The correct answer is "b."

Remission of diabetes after surgery is dependent on beta cell function. C-Peptide measurements especially when calculated in relation to glucose tolerance test (AUC), has been found to be more useful in prediction of diabetes remission after bariatric surgery.

Souteiro, P., Belo, S., Neves, J. S., Magalhães, D., Silva, R. B., Oliveira, S. C., . . . Carvalho, D. (2016, July 19). Preoperative Beta Cell Function Is Predictive of Diabetes Remission After Bariatric Surgery. Retrieved December 29, 2017, from https://link.springer.com/article/10.1007/s11695-016-2300-3

Question 10.20

42-year-old female presents in ER with abdominal pain of one-day duration. She has nausea and vomiting. The patient had a bariatric procedure five years ago. She had a couple of similar episodes of acute pain in the past few months. A CT scan done in ER shows a swirl of the mesentery. An internal hernia is suspected. Which of the following statements regarding her clinical condition is correct?

a. Immediate EGD is needed to evaluate the cause of pain

b. She likely had a sleeve gastrectomy surgery done in the past

c. She probably had a Roux-en-Y type gastric bypass surgery

d. The incidence of small bowel obstruction in post Sleeve Gastrectomy patients is similar to Roux-en-Y gastric bypass cases

e. Most cases of an internal hernia after gastric bypass with pain can be best managed with non-operative measures including nasogastric decompression, iv fluids and keeping patient nothing by mouth.

The correct answer is "c."

Internal hernias occur due to abnormal spaces and holes created after Roux-en-Y gastric bypass. These hernias are seen at jejunojejunostomy site and behind the Roux limb. The retrocolic version of gastric bypass is more vulnerable to the later type. This is also commonly known as Petersen's hernia. A high index of suspicion is required to identify this problem. Prompt surgical intervention can save bowel form ischemia. Radiological signs can be equivocal. Twist and swirling of mesentery may be noted on a CT scan. A negative CT scan does not rule out an internal hernia.

Lockhart, M. E., Tessler, F. N., Canon, C. L., Smith, J. K., Larrison, M. C., Fineberg, N. S., . . . Clements, R. H. (2007). Internal Hernia After Gastric Bypass: Sensitivity and Specificity of Seven CT Signs with Surgical Correlation and Controls. American Journal of Roentgenology, 188(3), 745-750. doi:10.2214/ajr.06.0541

Question 10.21

A 35-year-old female had an adjustable band placed a few years ago. She has developed pain and mild redness at the port access site for the last few days. She has a low-grade fever and intermittent nausea. Which of the following statements is correct regarding her clinical condition?

a. Erosion of band is a likely possibility

b. Gastrografin should be injected into the access port for further evaluation.

c. Removal of the band and concurrent conversion to sleeve gastrectomy should be considered

d. Emptying the band with oral antibiotics will likely resolve her symptom

e. Upper GI endoscopy is not helpful in diagnosing erosion.

The correct answer is "a."

An inflammatory response at the access port site is highly suggestive of band erosion and infection. Port access site infection can also happen once fill adjustments are performed. An EGD may show band erosion. This condition requires band removal. In acute infective conditions, conversion to sleeve gastrectomy should be avoided.

Juodeikis, %., Abalikšta, T., Brimiene, V., & Brimas, G. (2016). Laparoscopic Adjustable Gastric Banding: A Prospective Randomized Clinical Trial Comparing 5-Year Results of two Different Bands in 103 Patients. Obesity Surgery, 27(4), 1024-1030. doi:10.1007/s11695-016-2416-5

Question 10.22

A 30-year-old female who is status post-RYGB for morbid obesity presents in the emergency room with acute and severe upper abdominal pain. She is 25 weeks gravida. She had continuous nausea and vomited a few times since last night. Imaging with CT scan shows gas shadows in the small bowel. She has WBC of 12.5. Other labs including electrolytes are in normal range. There are no other specific findings. Which of the following statements is correct?

a. After giving pain medications, she may be discharged home
b. An internal hernia is the least likely diagnosis
c. A barium meal follow through study should be ordered.
d. She is at substantial risk of having complications related to her pregnancy including premature birth of the fetus
e. Majority of patients suspected to have an internal hernia after gastric bypass can be managed conservatively with nasogastric decompression, IV fluids and analgesics

The correct answer is "d."

Pregnancy in patients with RYGBP can have several challenges. In situations of acute abdomen, there can be high risks related to pregnancy. Any case suspected to have an internal hernia needs prompt intervention to avoid bowel ischemia. It is not appropriate to discharge such a patient.

Petersen, L., Lauenborg, J., Svare, J., & Nilas, L. (2016). The Impact of Upper Abdominal Pain During Pregnancy Following a Gastric Bypass. Obesity Surgery,27(3), 688-693. doi:10.1007/s11695-016-2339-1

Question 10.23

A 40-year-old male is experiencing daily symptoms of hypoglycemia. He had Roux-en-Y gastric bypass several years ago for morbid obesity. Which of the following statements is not correct about post-RYGBP hypoglycemia?

a. Extreme, progressive, unrecognized neuroglycopenic symptoms of postprandial hyperinsulinemic hypoglycemia can result in cognitive and neurologic impairment with the risk of seizures and loss of consciousness posing a risk to both the patient and others.

b. Diagnosis of postprandial hyperinsulinemic hypoglycemia requires a dietary journal, along with confirmatory laboratory and provocative testing, in the setting of symptoms presenting more than one year after surgery.

c. Postprandial hyperinsulinemic hypoglycemia cannot be effectively treated in most of the cases with dietary modification alone.

d. Pharmacotherapy produces variable results but should be attempted before surgical intervention. A gastrostomy tube with feeding into the excluded stomach provides nutritional support and, in some cases, symptomatic relief and should be considered in patients not responding to nonoperative treatment.

e. Insulinoma must be ruled out in patients with confirmed fasting hypoglycemia.

The correct answer is "c."

Most case of post gastric bypass hypoglycemia can be treated with dietary modifications. All the rest of the statements are correct.

Eisenberg, D., Azagury, D. E., Ghiassi, S., Grover, B. T., & Kim, J. J. (2017). ASMBS Position Statement on Postprandial Hyperinsulinemic Hypoglycemia after Bariatric Surgery. Surgery for Obesity and Related Diseases, 13(3), 371-378. doi: 10.1016/j.soard.2016.12.005

Question 10.24

Roux-en-Y gastric bypass (RYGBP) is known to have blood pressure lowering effect along with weight loss in obese patients. Which of the following statements is correct?

a. Excretion of renal sodium is decreased after RYGBP
b. Excretion of renal sodium is unaffected after RYGBP
c. Excretion of renal sodium Is increased after RYGBP
d. NT-proBNP (N-terminal pro b-type natriuretic peptide) levels are increased after RYGBP
e. Statements c and d are correct
f. None of the statements is correct

The correct answer is "e."

Renal fractional excretion of sodium is increased after RYGB. Increased postoperative basal and meal associated levels of NT-proBNP are observed. This is associated with increased urinary sodium excretion. This may be contributory to blood pressure lowering effects of the procedure.

Docherty, N. G., Fändriks, L., Roux, C. W., Hallersund, P., & Werling, M. (2017). Urinary sodium excretion after gastric bypass surgery. Surgery for Obesity and Related Diseases, 13(9), 1506-1514. doi: 10.1016/j.soard.2017.04.002

Question 10.25

The recommended minimum daily amount of Vitamin D3 (Cholecalciferol) after bariatric surgery is

a. 400 international units
b. 800 international units
c. 100 international units
d. 3000 international units

The correct answer is "d."

Question 10.26

DVT (Deep venous thrombosis) in obese patients, remains as one of the most feared complications after bariatric surgery. Various strategies are used to prevent DVT in bariatric patients in the perioperative period. Please select the correct statement.

a. Therapeutic effect of low molecular weight heparins can be assessed by anti-factor Xa activity.
b. Therapeutic effect of low molecular weight heparins can be assessed by anti-factor IXa activity.
c. Enoxaparin achieves acceptable anti-factor Xa levels in more than 90 percent of cases when given in a dose of 40 mg twice daily.
d. Magnetic resonance venography is used commonly to detect DVT in lower extremities.
e. Lower extremity venography is easy to perform in morbidly obese patients

The correct answer is “a."

Low molecular weight heparin assay (therapeutic range of 0.5 to 1 IU/ml) can be helpful in morbidly obese patients who receive enoxaparin for DVT prophylaxis. The dose can be adjusted according to the results. Studies have shown that a fair number of patients achieve less than optimal prophylaxis in the post-operative period.
“Enoxaparin Clinical Pearl.” Heart Failure, www.clevelandclinicmeded.com/medicalpubs/pharmacy/janfeb2003/enoxaparin.htm.

Question 10.27

A morbidly obese patient undergoes a bariatric procedure a couple of years ago. Her family physician requests a follow up with her bariatric surgeon for disturbing GERD symptoms. PPIs and Carafate were not helpful. She is investigated for her symptoms of heartburn and pain in the lower chest. Which of the following studies will not be of much help to evaluate and quantify GERD symptoms?

a. Upper GI endoscopy
b. Barium Swallow study for upper GI
c. Magnetic resonance cholangiopancreatography (MRCP) to check bile reflux to the stomach
d. Bravo study

The correct answer is "c."

In this case, upper GI study, barium swallow and Bravo capsule studies will be helpful. Considering the symptoms, MRCP will be of limited help. MRCP is useful for biliary system evaluation. Similarly, the gastric emptying study is not meant to see the severity of gastroesophageal reflux.

Question 10.28

Bravo study was done for the case mentioned above. The result reveals the following values. Acid exposure time (%) 22 (Normal < 4.9), Longest reflux 79 minutes, DeMeester score 84. Which of the following statements is correct?

a. Roux- en- Y gastric bypass is the likely bariatric procedure done for her
b. Sleeve gastrectomy is a more likely bariatric procedure done for her
c. From the numbers given, it is evident that she has mild reflux
d. The numbers stated does not reveal any reflux issue
e. Predominantly bile reflux is suspected

The correct answer is "b."

Sleeve gastrectomy is associated with gastroesophageal reflux more commonly. High DeMeester score confirms the presence of significant acid reflux. Normal DeMeester score should be < 14.7. Gastric bypass operation creates a small pouch with potentially a small amount of acid production with fewer chances of GERD. Gastric band and duodenal switch operations may also be associated with reflux symptoms.

Question 10.29

A 55-year-old female is seeking bariatric surgical option for weight loss. She has a history of DVT of the right lower extremity with PE at age of 39. Precipitating event at that time was the use of oral contraceptives. She is currently not on any anticoagulation. She is concerned and fearful about DVT developing again after bariatric surgery. She discusses her concerns with her family physician. Her risk assessment for DVT can be done by which of the following scoring systems?

a. Caprini's scoring system
b. APACHE II scoring system
c. American college of surgeon's surgical risk calculator
d. SAPS II scoring system

The correct answer is "a."

The validity of Caprini's scoring system in the assessment of DVT risk has been done in recent publications. This scoring system categorizes the risk as very low, low, moderate, and high based on the scores obtained. Recommendations about post-operative prophylaxis can be made based on the risk assessed. Monitoring is recommended for patients with very high weight (>150 kg). Anti-factor Xa is desired to be measured, and an acceptable level is believed to be 0.2 to 0.5 units/ml for unfractionated heparin (UH) and 0.5 to 1.0 for low molecular weight heparin (LMWH). Readers should be aware about some variability of therapeutic ranges and recommendations.

Dang, Jerry T., et al. "Predicting Venous Thromboembolism Following Laparoscopic Bariatric Surgery: Development of the

BariClot Tool Using the MBSAQIP Database." SpringerLink, Humana Press, 12 July 2018, link.springer.com/article/10.1007/s00464-018-6348-0.

Question 10.30

A 42-year-old female with morbid obesity with problems of DM2, HTN, Hyperlipidemia opts for Roux-en-Y gastric bypass surgery for weight loss. Her pre-operative BMI was 52. She had two C-Sections in past. Preoperative sonogram of the abdomen shows fatty liver. Gallbladder was normal. She lost about 45 pounds in four months after her bariatric procedure. She presents in the emergency department with an acute right upper quadrant abdominal pain. She is currently taking her medications for HTN, diabetes, oral multivitamins, and iron. She has a WBC count of 13.1, K 3.8, AST 101, ALT 92, and total bilirubin is 3.7 with a direct bilirubin level of 2.1. Please select the correct statement.

a. Rapid weight loss has no contribution to the development of her acute condition
b. Gallbladder disorder is an unlikely pathology
c. An ultrasound of right upper quadrant will be an initial investigation of choice in her case
d. Common bile duct on sonogram will be unlikely to be dilated due to gastric bypass status.
e. An ERCP (endoscopic retrograde cholangiopancreatography) through the mouth can resolve her issue

The correct answer is "c."

Question 10.31

In relation to preventions and management of the problem stated in the above question, select the correct statement

a. Calcium chloride has been proven to prevent the formation of gallstones
b. Occurrence of cholesterol and bile pigment gallstones can be completely prevented with the use of bile acid products
c. Ursodeoxycholic acid is a cholesterol-lowering agent
d. Removal of the gallbladder is practiced by most surgeons to prevent gallstone complications following gastric bypass surgery
e. Patient may likely need cholecystectomy and an ERCP (endoscopic retrograde cholangiopancreatography) through the excluded stomach with operative access.

The correct answer is "e."

Gallstones and acute gallbladder conditions may occur at a slightly higher frequency following rapid weight loss, especially after bariatric surgical procedures. Mobilization of cholesterol and other lipids contribute to the development of this condition. Prophylactic removal of an otherwise normal gallbladder is not a universally accepted option in most centers. Studies have shown the reduction of gallstone incidence by approximately 1/3rd with use of bile acid products following bariatric surgery. The incidence of gallstone formation is higher in the initial 6 months following bariatric surgery. It has also been noted that compliance for bile acid products like ursodeoxycholic acid is poor to fair in general due to side effects. Calcium chloride may help prevent formation of renal oxalate stones. Renal stone may form at higher frequency after gastric bypass due to altered calcium and fatty acid metabolism due to malabsorption component of gastric bypass.

Sattaratnamai, A., et al. "Gallstone Formation and Subsequent Cholecystectomy after Bariatric Surgery: A Systematic Review." Hpb, vol. 18, 2016, doi:10.1016/j.hpb.2016.03.375.

Question 10.32

A patient is planning for sleeve gastrectomy for morbid obesity. She is also planning a procedure for her foot related to a painful heel spur. It is expected that she will need a cast after her foot procedure. How long she should wait to get her second surgery after her bariatric procedure?

a. She can have her heel surgery immediately after her bariatric surgery
b. She should wait for a week before her second surgery
c. She should wait for 6 months before her heel surgery
d. She does <u>not</u> carry higher chances of deep venous thrombosis if she gets the heel spur surgery sooner due to immobilization of her foot and decreased activity.
e. It would be best to wait for at least few months before any elective surgery after bariatric procedure. It may also be determined on case-by-case basis depending on the urgency. Adequate precautions and prophylaxis for deep venous thrombosis should be done if decreased activity is expected.

The correct answer is "e."

Question 10.33

A patient is preparing for her bariatric surgery. She has been a smoker for several years. She recently quit smoking. She has bronchial asthma and uses bronchodilators as needed. She is advised to see a pulmonologist for preoperative evaluation. She undergoes pulmonary function testing. Pulmonologist authors a detailed report and sends a copy to the bariatric surgeon and another to her family physician. He uses a point system to describe risk stratification for her. Which of the following scoring systems can be used for an objective preoperative pulmonary assessment?

a. ARISCAT risk index
b. APGAR scoring system
c. Ranson's criteria
d. Child-Pugh scoring system

Correct answer is "a."
ARISCAT system is used for pulmonary risk stratification. It looks at oxygen saturation, surgical incision location and expected length of surgery. A score between 0 and 25 points predicts 1.6 % risk of pulmonary complications. A score between 45 and 123 predicts 42.1% risk of postoperative complications. Morbidly obese patients have a higher score due to presence of sleep apnea, restrictive lung disease, longer duration of surgery and upper abdominal incisions. APGAR score is done for newborns. Ranson's criteria are used in pancreatitis. Child's scoring system is used for liver disease.

Question 10.34

A patient is considering bariatric surgery for morbid obesity. He has heart burn symptoms for some time Please select the correct statement.

a. Diagnosis of eosinophilic esophagitis is confirmed
b. Eosinophilic esophagitis presence is a contraindication for gastric bypass
c. Eosinophilic esophagitis is a contraindication for sleeve gastrectomy
d. This condition reflects allergy to some food items, and it is not an absolute contraindication for bariatric surgery

Correct answer is "d."

The condition is thought to result from allergic reaction to various antigenic stimuli. Symptoms may vary and include heartburn, abdominal pain, regurgitation of food, and dysphagia. Presence of eosinophilic esophagitis is not an absolute contraindication to weight loss surgery. More than 15 eosinophils per high power field confirms the diagnosis of eosinophilic esophagitis.

Question 10.35

Alcohol use disorder (AUD) in patients seeking bariatric surgery needs careful attention. In some patients, this may become a concerning issue in the post-operative phase. Please select the correct statement.

a. Females are more likely to suffer from this disorder than males
b. Patient undergoing gastric band are more likely to suffer from this disorder than patients who had Roux-en-Y gastric bypass.
c. Smokers and those addicted to other recreational drugs are less prone to have alcohol use disorder
d. Incidence of this disorder is higher in the second postoperative year than first one
e. Major site of production of alcohol dehydrogenase is the colon

Correct answer is "d."

In post gastric bypass setting, peak blood level of alcohol is reached earlier. Plasma clearance of alcohol is also delayed. In gastric bypass patients this may also contribute to faster absorption. Females are not more likely to suffer from AUD compared to males. Alcohol use disorder is more likely after gastric bypass compared to gastric banding. Patients with history of other addictions are more likely to suffer from AUD. Stomach and not the colon is the site contributing to major production of alcohol dehydrogenase.

J.C. Hagedorn, B. Encarnacion, G.A. Brat, J.M. Morton Does gastric bypass alter alcohol metabolism? Surg Obes Relat Dis, 3 (5) (2007), pp. 543–548

Question 10.36

A 50-year-old male with BMI 58 weighing 370 lb undergoes a conversion surgery from sleeve gastrectomy to a Roux-en-Y bypass due to failure to lose weight. Surgery was difficult due to adhesions related to previous abdominal procedures. The procedure took more than 4 hours. A panel of labs was done in recovery room. It showed serum creatinine 2.1 mg/dl. His preoperative value was 0.9 mg/dl. He had a Foley's catheter in place and urine output is low. Select the correct statement.

a. Dehydration is unlikely to be a cause for his condition
b. A dose of dexamethasone given during surgery as part of ERAS (Enhanced recovery after surgery) protocol could have caused the condition
c. Creatine level goes up after most bariatric surgery procedures
d. Muscle cell damage with increased intracellular free ionized calcium in cytoplasm and mitochondria is a likely reason

Correct answer is "d."
The description in the question points to rhabdomyolysis. An increase in intracellular free ionized calcium in cytoplasm and mitochondria is the final common pathway after injury to the muscle fibers. ATP depletion or cell membrane damage can lead to that. Muscle enzymes including creatine kinase (CK) is released. This condition requires aggressive management with IV fluids and forced diuresis to prevent renal failure. Dehydration can lead to acute rise in creatinine, but possibility of rhabdomyolysis should be kept in mind and ruled out for

procedures longer than 4 hours. Dexamethasone injection is not likely to cause acute rise in creatinine. Acute elevation of creatinine after bariatric surgery is not common and should be investigated and treated.

Question 10.37

A 30-year-old female patient wants to lose weight. She has a current BMI of 36. She is afraid of undergoing bariatric surgery as one of her family members had complications after gastric bypass surgery. She read an article in one of the health magazines about intragastric balloons. She wants to learn more about this option. Please select the correct statement.

a. Intragastric balloons can help with a loss of 40 to 50% of excess weight.
b. Intragastric balloons cause weight loss through malabsorption.
c. A laparoscopic procedure is needed for placement of intragastric balloons.
d. Previous gastric surgery, coagulation disorder, pregnancy, alcoholism or other addiction, liver disease and the presence of any contraindications for upper endoscopy are absolute contraindications for intragastric balloons.

Correct answer is "d."

Weight loss with intragastric balloons is in the range of 5 to 10% of excess weight. As of 2019, most health insurance plans in the United States do not cover this procedure. It is a temporary method of weight loss. The balloons can be left in place for 6 months at a time. Proposed mechanism of weight loss is restriction of food intake and not the malabsorption. Upper endoscopy is needed for placement and removal of some intragastric balloons (Orbera Intragastric balloon). Laparoscopic procedure is not needed for placement or removal of any intragastric balloons. One of the intragastric balloons currently available in USA can be ingested orally and does not need endoscopy for placement but does need upper endoscopy for removal (Obalon intragastric balloon). Contraindications are as stated in option "d."

Question 10.38

A hospital in US is looking into intragastric balloon procedures to expand its bariatric surgery program. Pros and cons are discussed in a meeting with the administration. As most health insurance plans are not covering this procedure as of 2019, the patients will be paying cash for this procedure. Hospital CEO wants to know the risks especially readmissions to factor out the costs. What is the most common reason for readmission for patients undergoing intragastric balloon?

a. Gastric bleed
b. Small bowel obstruction
c. Balloon failure due to rupture
d. Nausea, vomiting, pain and dehydration

Correct answer is "d."

The most common reason for readmission after intragastric balloon insertion is nausea, vomiting, dehydration and abdominal pain. Most of the time it can be managed with antiemetics and iv hydration. Small number of cases may require admission for hydration, pain, and nausea control.

Question 10.39

Aspire assist® is an FDA approved option for weight loss for some patients. Please select the correct statement about this modality.

a. A nasogastric tube is placed for aspiration of stomach contents
b. It is meant for long term use only
c. It is approved for pediatric patients
d. Food should not be chewed well for this therapy to be successful.

Correct answer is "b."

Aspire assist® device is placed with endoscopic or laparoscopic assistance in the stomach. It is FDA approved in adults of age 22 or older for patients with BMI of 35 to 55 if they have failed to lose weight with diet and lifestyle modifications. Patients need to chew food well and should be able to aspirate the contents of the stomach using this device (Average is 2.5 times daily). Lifestyle therapy is continuously needed.

Question 10.40

A 59-year-old patent is referred to a bariatric practice for consideration of weight loss surgery. He smoked for 40 years and has severe COPD. He uses a motorized scooter to get around and uses 2 liters/minute of oxygen all the time. Please select the correct statement about his risk and feasibility for bariatric surgery.

a. Laparoscopic gastric bypass could be the safest option
b. He can undergo bariatric surgery with lower complications but higher mortality risks
c. He can undergo bariatric surgery with higher complications but less mortality risks
d. He can undergo bariatric surgery with higher complications but similar mortality risks

Correct answer is "d."

Retrospective data points toward the fact that oxygen dependent patient can undergo bariatric surgery with higher complications but similar mortality risks. Sleeve gastrectomy may be a safer option than gastric bypass surgery for patients with oxygen dependency.

Question 10.41

Roux-en-Y Gastric bypass surgery alters incretin effect. Please select the correct statement.

a. RYGBP decrease the incretin effect
b. RYGBP restores the incretin effect
c. Incretin effect is increased by several folds in obese patients with type 2 diabetes
d. IV glucose administration leads to the production of more insulin compared to oral glucose administration.

Correct answer is "b."

Incretin effect is the reason for release of more insulin if glucose is taken orally as compared to IV administration. GLP1 and GIP are thought to be responsible for this effect. Incretin effect is decreased or absent in patients with type 2 diabetes.

Question 10.42

Early dumping is a well-known issue in gastric bypass patients. Please select the correct statement about this condition.

a. Hyperosmolar contents entering from stomach pouch to small bowel cause early dumping syndrome
b. Shift of fluid from intravascular to bowel lumen space leads to some of the vasomotor effects.

c. It occurs half to one hour after meals
d. Early dumping improves in most patients over time with dietary modifications
e. All the above statements are correct

Correct answer is "e."

Question 10.43

Select the correct statement about neuroglycopenia.

a. It is due to reduced glycogen production by the liver
b. It leads to 'passing out' or fainting due to low blood sugar level
c. GLP1 agonists are helpful in the treatment
d. Insulinoma is a common entity in patients with history of RYGBP

Correct answer is "b."

Neuroglycopenia is a relatively less common complication after gastric bypass. It is different from dumping syndrome as it occurs later. It is difficult to treat in most cases. Its etiology is multifactorial. Nesidioblastosis is considered in the differential diagnosis. Options for its treatment include dietary changes (reduction in intake of refined carbohydrates and increasing intake of proteins, frequent small meals) and pharmacotherapy.

Hypoglycemia After Gastric Bypass Surgery
Ekta Singh, Adrian Vella
Diabetes Spectrum Nov 2012, 25 (4) 217-221; DOI: 10.2337/diaspect.25.4.217

Question 10.44

A patient had RYGBP surgery 5 years ago. She is suffering from recurrent attacks of hypoglycemia. She is referred to an endocrinology practice for evaluation. As part of the work up, the endocrinologist plans for 72 hours fasting test. Please select the correct answer

a. This test is likely to be positive in the case of nesidioblastosis
b. This test is likely to be negative in dumping syndrome
c. It is likely to be negative in insulinoma
d. All the above statements are correct

Correct answer is "b."

72 hours fasting test is negative in dumping syndrome and nesidioblastosis. It is positive in cases of insulinoma. Hypoglycemia may be a challenging condition to treat after gastric bypass. Portion control with diets of low glycemic index, use of somatostatin analogues, diazoxide or calcium channel blockers may be helpful. Some patients may need gastric tube feeding. Various other surgical options like partial/subtotal pancreatectomy, reversal of gastric bypass or

other modifications of the Roux-en- Y configuration of gastric bypass may be considered.

Question 10.45

Osteoporosis risk increases after weight loss surgery. Which one of the following procedures has the highest risk of causing osteoporosis?

a. Adjustable gastric band
b. Sleeve gastrectomy
c. Roux-en-Y gastric bypass
d. Intragastric balloon

Correct answer is "c."
Gastric bypass patients have higher risk of developing osteoporosis compared to sleeve gastrectomy and adjustable gastric banding. Vitamin D and calcium deficiencies can contribute to this. Patients are recommended to stay on lifelong supplementation of calcium and vitamin D. Levels of Vitamin D 25 hydroxy, PTH and calcium should be monitored closely.

Question 10.46

A patient with remote history of gastric bypass had a DEXA scan for bone density assessment. Her family physician wants to consider bisphosphonate therapy. He would like to have input from her bariatric surgeon for any risks with its use. A letter is sent to the bariatric surgery office for input regarding this issue. What is the risk in gastric bypass patients with use of this medicine?

a. Cardiac arrythmia
b. Marginal ulcers
c. Insomnia
d. Weight gain

Correct answer is “b.”

Evidence based recommendations for use of antiresorptive therapy in bariatric patients are lacking. Use of oral bisphosphonates in bariatric surgery patients is associated with increased risk of marginal ulcers and severe reflux. Some authors may consider IV therapy if vitamin D level is normal. Hypocalcemia with tetany may be observed in patient who have vitamin D and calcium deficiencies. There may be higher risk of fractures with use of bisphosphonates.

Stein, Emily M, and Shonni J Silverberg. “Bone loss after bariatric surgery: causes, consequences, and management.” *The lancet. Diabetes & endocrinology* vol. 2,2 (2014): 165-74. doi:10.1016/S2213-8587(13)70183-9

Question 10.47

A 55-year-old male had gastric bypass surgery 10 years ago. His preoperative BMI was 58 and he weighed 275 lbs. His lowest weight was 166 lbs., and it was achieved after two years of surgery. He has experienced weight gain in the last 3 years. His current weight is 225 lbs. He is very concerned. His family physician has started his diabetic medications again and has added a diuretic for uncontrolled hypertension. Please select the correct statement regarding his condition.

a. 20 to 30 % patients experience significant weight regain after gastric bypass surgery
b. In most patients, poor eating habits contribute to weight regain
c. Gastrogastric fistula, dilated gastric pouch and stretched gastrojejunal anastomosis could contribute to weight regain after Roux-en-Y gastric bypass
d. Alcohol use disorder could contribute to significant weight regain after Roux-en-Y gastric bypass.
e. All above statements are correct

Correct answer is "e."

Bariatric surgery is the most effective treatment for morbid obesity. Majority of the patients can maintain most of the weight lost after bariatric surgery. However, some patients do experience weight regain over long term. The correct figure is in the range of 20 to 30% for weight recidivism after Roux-en-Y gastric bypass procedure.

Question 10.48

A morbidly obese patient seeking bariatric surgery is getting ready for the procedure in a few weeks. She is concerned about post-operative nausea. She had gallbladder surgery a couple of years ago with a very rough postoperative course. She has read an article in a health magazine about ERAS (enhanced recovery after surgery). She wants to learn more about ERAS related to bariatric surgery. Please select the correct statement about ERAS.

a. Preoperative carbohydrate loading may have beneficial affect
b. Avoiding administration of excessive IV fluids during anesthesia helps in quicker recovery
c. Laparoscopic /minimal invasive surgery enhances recovery
d. Minimizing use of narcotics is recommended
e. All the above statements are correct

Correct answer is "e."

Enhanced recovery after surgery (ERAS) is a rapidly growing concept in most surgical disciplines. It focuses on optimization of comorbidities, use of multimodal analgesia, better control of post-operative nausea and vomiting, better control of blood sugar and goal directed fluid administration. Optimization of these factors leads to enhanced recovery and potentially prevent some complications and shortens the hospital stay.

Question 10.49

A post gastric bypass patient who is currently a smoker follows with a bariatric practice. She smokes a pack daily. She has developed marginal ulcers in the past and had one incidence of marginal ulcer perforation requiring laparoscopic repair. An attempt to quit smoking in past caused her to gain weight. Bariatric surgeon is working closely with family physician to help her stop smoking. A decision is made to check her biochemistry randomly for compliance for nonsmoking. Please select the correct statement.

a. Nicotine half-life is about 0.5 to 3 hours and for Continine it is about 16 to 19 hours
b. Tobacco cigarette and "vaping" e-cigarettes produce similar level of continine
c. Gastric bypass status does not alter the pharmacokinetics or dynamics of nicotine
d. Stopping smoking frequently results in weight gain
e. All above statements are correct

Correct answer is "e."

Statements (a) to (d) are correct. Continine level is the preferred test to check for tobacco use and compliance for nonsmoking. Some of the other short-lived metabolites used to check for smoking status include anabasine and nornicotine. Nicotine does carry a suppressant effect on appetite. Smoking increases the risk of developing and non-healing of marginal ulcers.

Question 10.50

What is the incidence of relapse of type 2 diabetes after bariatric surgery?

a. 5%
b. 20%

c. 50%
d. 75%

Correct answer is "c."

Bariatric surgery is extremely effective for remission of type 2 diabetes in short term. However about 50% of patients experience a relapse of diabetes within 10 years' time. Older patients with a prolonged history of diabetes and poor control have higher risk of relapse.

Question 10.51

Various scoring systems are used to predict remission of diabetes after Roux-en-Y gastric bypass. Which one of the following scoring systems is found to be useful in this respect?

a. Diarem scoring system
b. Child's scoring system
c. Mallampati classification system
d. DeMeester scoring system

The correct answer is "a."

Diarem scoring system is found to be reliable in predicting remission of diabetes type 2 after various bariatric procedures. Child scoring system is used to assess severity of liver disease. Mallampati systems is used for upper airway assessment especially before anesthesia. DeMeester scoring is dedicated to quantifying GERD symptoms.

Question 10.52

A morbidly obese patient is getting investigated before her planned sleeve gastrectomy procedure. An EGD as part of preoperative workup shows moderate amount of food in the stomach. She is advised to have a gastric emptying study for a suspected diagnosis of gastroparesis. A dual phase gastric emptying study is done few days later. It shows calculated T-½ solid phase of gastric emptying time of 105 minutes suggestive of mild gastroparesis. Normal range of gastric emptying is 60 to 90 minutes. Patient want to know what the T-1/2 means in the test report and whether her high BMI has an effect on the results. Please select the correct answer.

a. T ½ means half of lag time before gastric emptying starts
b. T ½ means the time it takes to empty half of stomach contents
c. BMI is found to have profound effect on gastric emptying
d. Female gender and phase of menstrual cycle have no effect on gastric emptying

The correct answer is "b."
T ½ relates to the time it takes for half of the stomach contents to empty. A range of factors which may affect gastric emptying include female gender, phase of menstrual cycle, position, time of day, BMI, and drinking alcohol. Smokers have shorter gastric emptying T ½ time. Efforts are made to standardize the gastric emptying study with various kinds of meals. Western and ascian meals have been tested on volunteers in this regard.

J Neurogastroenterol Motil. 2014 Jul; 20(3): 371–378.
doi: 10.5056/jnm13114

Vasavid P, Chaiwatanarat T, Pusuwan P, Sritara C, Roysri K, Namwongprom S, Kuanrakcharoen P, Premprabha T, Chunlertrith K, Thongsawat S, Sirinthornpunya S, Ovartlarnporn B, Kachintorn U, Leelakusolvong S, Kositchaiwat C, Chakkaphak S, Gonlachanvit S. Normal Solid Gastric Emptying Values Measured by Scintigraphy Using Asian-style Meal:A Multicenter Study in Healthy Volunteers. J Neurogastroenterol Motil. 2014 Jul 31;20(3):371-8. doi: 10.5056/jnm13114. PMID: 24948129; PMCID: PMC4102158.

Question 10.53

Adjustable gastric band was done for a patient with morbid obesity several years ago. She lost 45 lbs. in 12 months. She is now struggling with severe GERD symptoms. Her current BMI is 47. She is interested in revisional bariatric surgery. She opts for conversion to Roux-en-Y gastric bypass. Please select the correct statement.

a. Gastric bypass conversion from a sleeve gastrectomy, relieves GERD symptoms in all cases in addition to weight loss
b. Having previous gastric banding is risk factor for persistence of GERD symptoms after gastric bypass
c. She should have sleeve gastrectomy procedure instead
d. Single anastomosis duodenal switch would be a better option for her

The correct answer is "b."
Previous history of gastric adjustable band and symptoms of reflux is identified as a risk factor for the persistence of reflux symptoms after conversion to a Roux-en-Y configuration. Sleeve gastrectomy may not be a suitable option as is single anastomosis duodenal switch. Both procedures involve making a tube out of stomach with increased potential of GERD.

Conversion of sleeve gastrectomy to Roux -en-Y gastric bypass in patients with gastroesophageal reflux disease: results of a multicenter study
Surgery for Obesity and Related Disease 16(2020) 732-737

Question 10.54

A lot of emphasis is made on enhanced recovery after bariatric surgery. American College of Surgeons and American Society of Bariatric and metabolic surgery have taken initiatives in this regard. BSTOP protocol is introduced, and a large trial is designed.

a. BSTOP targets to optimize sleep apnea
b. BSTOP targets to optimize various vitamins before surgery
c. BSTOP targets to optimize narcotic medications
d. BSTOP mandated used of continuous basal patient-controlled analgesia (PCA) with morphine

The correct answer is "c."
BSTOP stands for Bariatric Surgery Targeting Opioid Prescriptions (BSTOP). Emphasis is to minimize opioid use in perioperative period. This helps in reducing post operative nausea and enhanced recovery.
https://www.facs.org/Quality-Programs/MBSAQIP/News/bstop

Question 10.55

Data from Metabolic and Bariatric Surgery Accreditation and Quality improvement was used in a study to check the 30-day morbidity and mortality in males and females after bariatric surgery. Please select the correct statement.

a. Male sex was found to be a risk factor for having more complications
b. Male sex was found to be risk factor for all-cause mortality in 30 days
c. Female sex was found to be a risk factor for all-cause mortality in 30 days
d. No difference between two sexes was found regarding 30-day mortality and complications

The correct answer is "b."
Male sex is risk factor for all-cause mortality in 30 days where has females have higher risk of complications.
Comment on: A comparison of short-term outcomes after Roux-en-Y gastric bypass in male and female patients using MBSAQIP
Laura E. Fischer, M.D., M.S.
Published: July 02, 2020DOI:https://doi.org/10.1016/j.soard.2020.06.012

Question 10.56

Various parameters can be used to predict diabetes remission after Roux-en-Y gastric bypass. Which one of the followings is <u>not</u> a parameter to predict remission of diabetes after Roux-en-Y gastric bypass?

a. Hepatic steatosis
b. C Peptide
c. Duration of diabetes
d. History of cholecystectomy

The correct answer is "d."
History of cholecystectomy is not a parameter to predict remission of diabetes. Options a, b and c have predictive role. History of cholecystectomy does have association with post operative hypoglycemia and dumping syndrome in setting of Roux-en-Y gastric bypass.

Presence of Liver Steatosis is Associated with greater diabetes remission after gastric bypass surgery

Roman Vangoitsenhoven MD PhD1,2, Rickesha Wilson MD1, Deepa V Cherla MD1, Sangeeta R Kashyap MD3, David E Cummings MD4, Philip R Schauer MD1, Ali Aminian MD1
1 Bariatric and Metabolic Institute, Cleveland Clinic, Cleveland, Ohio, USA
2 Department of Endocrinology, UZ Leuven, Leuven, Belgium
3 Endocrine and Metabolism Institute, Cleveland Clinic, Cleveland, Ohio, USA
4 VA Puget Sound Health Care System and UW Medicine Institute, University of Washington, Seattle, WA

Question 10.57

A physician assistant student is rotating with a bariatric practice. She wants to work in emergency medicine in future. During rounds the Bariatric surgeon asks student a question which refers to the most common reason bringing a patient with gastric adjustable band to visit emergency department. Please select the correct answer

a. Band erosion to the stomach
b. Internal hernia
c. Gastric outlet obstruction due to tight band or slip
d. GI bleeding

The correct answer is "c."
Gastric outlet obstruction remains as one of the common reasons to visit ER. Not infrequently after fill adjustment of band, patients may experience upper GI symptoms in the form of nausea, vomiting or dysphagia. GI bleeding is more common in patients with gastric bypass with marginal ulcers. Similarly internal hernias occur more frequently in patients with history of gastric bypass.

Question 10.58

A patient had Roux-en-Y gastric bypass surgery 12 years ago. She had several complications after surgery including several episodes of small bowel obstruction and development of incisional hernias. She required several open explorations of the abdomen requiring lysis of adhesions. Last surgery was 3 years ago. She has anorexia and chronic diarrhea ever since. She has a current weight of 75 lbs. with a BMI of 15. She is wheelchair bound. She was feeling very week and had significant edema of her lower extremities. She was sent to the hospital for admission for severe malnutrition after seeing in the office. Initial work up did not show any bowel obstruction. Gastroenterology service was consulted to place a nasal tube for feeding. Additionally, she is started on partial parenteral nutrition. Concerns are raised about refeeding syndrome. Please select the correct statement.

a. High phosphate levels are more likely to be seen
b. Low phosphate levels are more likely to be seen
c. Reason of developing refeeding syndrome is likely shift of metabolism form carbohydrates predominantly to proteins for energy
d. High magnesium and potassium would be a likely finding.

The correct answer is "b."
Refeeding syndrome can be a serious consequence once feeding is resumed after a period of severe malnutrition. Shift of metabolism from predominantly fats and proteins as source of energy to carbohydrates occurs. Expected electrolyte abnormalities could be low phosphate, magnesium, hypokalemia. Fluid overload, and sodium level abnormalities may also be observed. Symptoms of refeeding syndrome may include, confusion, altered mental status, weakness, seizures,

fatigue, shortness of breath, arrhythmias, and CHF. Risk of mortality is high. Thiamine replacement is needed. It is recommended that feeding should be gradually increased. Initial daily calories may be kept around 1000.
https://www.healthline.com/health/refeeding-syndrome

Question 10.59

Various tools have been explored in predicting remission of diabetes and as a prognostic parameter following bariatric surgery. Two of such indices used are Neutrophil-lymphocyte (NLR) and platelet to lymphocyte (PLR) ratios. Please select he correct statement.

a. PLR is found to be a more useful index in predicting remission of diabetes type 2 and weight loss before bariatric surgery
b. NLR is found be a more promising index in prediction of remission of diabetes type 2 and weight loss before bariatric surgery
c. Both PLR and NLR are useful in predicting remission of diabetes type 2 and weight loss before bariatric surgery
d. None of PLR and NLR ratios have been found to be useful in predicting remission of diabetes type and weight loss.

The correct answer is "b."
It is shown that lower preoperative NLR can fairly predict the potential remission of type 2 diabetes, glycemic control, and weight loss at 5 years.
ORIGINAL ARTICLE: SURGERY| VOLUME 16, ISSUE 8, P999-1004, AUGUST 01, 2020

Correlation of preoperative neutrophil-to-lymphocyte ratio and platelet-to-lymphocyte ratio with metabolic parameters in patients undergoing sleeve gastrectomy
Lorea Zubiaga, M.D., PhD
Jaime Ruiz-Tovar, M.D., Ph.D.

Question 10.60

Readmission after bariatric surgery has been seen as one of the "quality of care" parameters. Which one of the following can predict readmission in 30 days?

a. CRP value
b. Hemoglobin value
c. WBC count at discharge
d. Blood urea/creatinine ratio

The correct answer is "a."
CRP value <27 at day 1 after surgery has a 96.6% negative predictive value for readmission after bariatric surgery.

Pediatric Obesity

Question 11.1

Childhood obesity has increased to a concerning level in recent years. Which of the following statements is correct about the definition of this condition?

a. BMI at 65th percentile is regarded as obesity
b. BMI at 75th percentile is regarded as obesity
c. BMI at 85th percentile is regarded as obesity
d. BMI at 95th percentile or above is considered as obesity
e. BMI at 70th percentile or above is regarded as a risk for obesity

The correct answer is "d."

Children above 95% percentile are considered obese. Alternately body fat percentage can be used to define obesity in the pediatric age group. For boys over 25% and girls over 32% fat is considered as criteria for obesity. BMI exceeding 120% of the 95th percentile is considered severe obesity.

Barlow, S. E. (2007). Expert Committee Recommendations Regarding the Prevention, Assessment, and Treatment of Child and Adolescent Overweight and Obesity: Summary Report. Pediatrics, 120(Supplement 4). doi:10.1542/peds.2007-2329c

Question 11.2

A pediatrician has several patients in her practice who are struggling with weight issues. They are in different age groups and have various stages of Tanner's maturity. Which Tenner's group has the most urgency to treat obesity?

a. Tanner's maturity index of 1 with height at 60th percentile
b. Tanner's maturity index of 2 with open epiphysis of long bones
c. Tanner's maturity index of 3 with closed epiphysis of long bones
d. Tanner's maturity index of 3 with open epiphysis of long bones
e. Tanner's maturity index of 4 with closed epiphysis of long bones

The correct answer is "d."

Tanner's maturity index of 3 in an obese child with advanced bone age needs close attention to avoid growth issues due to premature closure of epiphysis. It is recommended to do X-ray studies to determine bone age if necessary.

Marshall, W. A., & Tanner, J. M. (1970). Variations in the Pattern of Pubertal Changes in Boys. Archives of Disease in Childhood, 45(239), 13-23. doi:10.1136/adc.45.239.13

Marshall, W. A., & Tanner, J. M. (1969). Variations in pattern of pubertal changes in girls. Archives of Disease in Childhood, 44(235), 291-303. doi:10.1136/adc.44.235.291

Question 11.3

Which of the following is the top source of added sugar in the age group under 18 years?

a. Sodas
b. Candy
c. Dairy Desserts
d. Grain Desserts
e. Fruit Drinks

The correct answer is "a."

Sweetened drinks remain as a top source of added sugar in under 18 age group.

Reedy, J., & Krebs-Smith, S. M. (2010). Dietary Sources of Energy, Solid Fats, and Added Sugars among Children and Adolescents in the United States. Journal of the American Dietetic Association, 110(10), 1477-1484. doi: 10.1016/j.jada.2010.07.010

Question 11.4

What is the most common syndromic obesity?

a. Cohen Syndrome
b. Prader-Willi Syndrome
c. Carpenter Syndrome
d. Bardet-Biedl Syndrome

The correct answer is "b."

Prader-Willi Syndrome remains as most common syndromic obesity

Question 11.5

Patients with Prader-Willi syndrome are typically characterized by which of the following features?

a. Hypotonia, feeding problems with failure to thrive in infants and toddlers
b. Voracious appetite, decreased cognition and hypogonadism in adolescents and adults
c. Short stature relative to the genetic background
d. All the above statements are correct

The correct answer is "d."

Short stature, increased appetite, hypogonadism, and cognition problems are features of Prader-Willi syndrome. In early life issues related to feeding and failure to thrive are observed

Question 11.6

Life-threatening conditions related to Prader- Willi syndrome include which of the following?

a. Diabetes Mellitus
b. Obstructive Sleep Apnea
c. Rupture of the stomach
d. All the above statements are correct

The correct answer is "d."

Question 11.7

Choose the INCORRECT statement regarding treatment options for Prader-Willi syndrome.

a. Treatment includes strictly limited access to food through close supervision
b. Creation of physical barriers to prevent access to food

c. Pharmacologic agents including phentermine, topiramate and their combination

d. Growth Hormone treatment may improve linear growth, body composition, and bone density abnormalities

The correct answer is "c."

Phentermine is not an approved drug under the age of 18.

Question 11.8

Which of the following is the single most effective intervention to achieve weight loss in a child?

a. Use of combination weight loss medications

b. Intensive exercise

c. Frequent fasting

d. Reducing the intake of sweetened beverages

e. No breakfast on most days

The correct answer is "d."

Question 11.9

There is evidence that adolescent girls who consume more proteins at breakfast consumed fewer calories per day. Which of the following is the best answer for expected fewer calories per day consumed for this group?

a. 100 calories

b. 200 calories

c. 300 calories

d. 400 calories

The correct answer is "d."

Question 11.10

Genetic factors can influence the development of obesity in the pediatric age group. Genetic testing can be helpful to detect some of the related disorders. In which group of pediatric patients, it may be useful to suggest this kind of testing.?

a. 18-year-old female who likes ice creams and cookies and has a BMI of 35

b. A 12-year-old male child with BMI at 99th percentile and whose mother has a duodenal switch. Mother takes the child to a nearby fast-food chain after school for burgers and soda

c. A 4-year-old girl with BMI at 97th percentile and has dysmorphic facial features.

d. A 5-year-old boy who has a BMI at 95 th percentile. He has hyperphagia and has a brother who is seven years old. Brother's BMI is at the 98th percentile

e. "c." and "d." are correct statements.

The correct answer is "e."

Pediatric Obesity—Assessment, Treatment, and Prevention ... academic.oup.com/jcem/article/102/3/709/2965084.

Question 11.11

Diagnosing diabetes has been an issue in pediatric obesity. Select the correct statement regarding HbA1c levels in pediatric patients?

a. HbA1c has proved to be a reliable method of diagnosing diabetes in pediatric patients.

b. HbA1c is a cost-effective method in screening obese pediatric patients for diabetes and prediabetes

c. HbA1c value is not significantly affected by racial and ethnic variations

d. Fasting, random blood sugar or standard glucose tolerance test are more reliable tests to predict diabetes.

e. 2-hour glucose tolerance test is about 50% effective in diagnosing diabetes

The correct answer is "d."

HbA1c is not an ideal test for diagnosing diabetes in children. Ethnic and racial variations exist. 2-hour glucose tolerance test is a sensitive test. Fasting blood sugar of equal to or more than 126 mg /dl, and two-hour glucose equal to or more than 200 mg /dl, random glucose value of equal to or more than 200mg /dl and an A1C level of 6.5% or more are diagnostic criteria per ADA 2000 CS.

Pediatric Obesity—Assessment, Treatment, and Prevention academic.oup.com/jcem/article/102/3/709/2965084.

Question 11.12

Bariatric surgery is increasingly considered for adolescent patients. Significant progress has been made in the recent years in defining and compiling guidelines based on available evidence. Please select the correct statement.

a. Adolescents have shown better resolution of diabetes after bariatric surgery than adult patients.
b. A multidisciplinary team approach is needed once adolescents are considered for bariatric surgery
c. A long-term follow-up plan is a key to better outcomes
d. It is determined that more than two third of adolescent patients are not compliant with vitamins and other nutritional supplements after two years of their surgery
e. All the above statements are correct

The correct answer is "e."

Bariatric surgery for morbidly obese adolescents is performed more frequently now at dedicated bariatric surgery centers. Bariatric surgery is effective for weight loss, treatment, and prevention of weight related comorbidities in this group. A multidisciplinary approach is required with long-term follow up strategies. Published data reflects lower morbidity for this group of patients compared to adults. Long term compliance with vitamins and other nutritional supplements continues to be a challenge in this group of patients.

Pediatric Obesity—Assessment, Treatment, and Prevention ... academic.oup.com/jcem/article/102/3/709/2965084.

Question 11.13

A mother brings her son to a bariatric office for consultation for weight gain. He is a 14-year-old 8th grade student. His BMI is at the 99th percentile for his age. The 6-year-old younger sister of the patient has also accompanied the family. Both kids are holding bags of French fries and large glasses of regular sodas. Mother had a duodenal switch 12 years ago. She does two jobs and has no time for cooking. She often buys fast food for the kids. "French fries" is an item in most meals. She wants duodenal switch operation for her son and appears very concerned about his health and weight gain. She also mentioned the boy being bullied and teased at school because of his weight.

a. Duodenal switch operation should be offered to the patient as it is one of the most powerful operations for weight loss.

b. Doing duodenal switch will compensate for some of the eating patterns which exist

c. The child should be started on bupropion and naltrexone combination right away

d. Bariatric surgery should be offered to the child as a primary option at its earliest as he is at risk of developing diabetes and sleep apnea.

e. Multidisciplinary team efforts are needed for the education of mother, family, and the patient. Healthy diet and physical activity are two of the important components of such efforts. Bariatric surgery does not seem to be an appropriate choice in the current situation.

The correct answer is "e."

Here the health care provider is facing a challenging situation. A lot of counseling is needed. Mother has a great responsibillty on her shoulders. Her intentions are not matching her actions. An evaluation for readiness to change the situation is essential in this scenario.

Pediatric Obesity—Assessment, Treatment, and Prevention academic.oup.com/jcem/article/102/3/709/2965084.

Question 11.14

A 19-year-old girl is diagnosed with polycystic ovaries. She has a BMI of 39. She has irregular periods. Lab work shows insulin resistance with elevated levels. She is started on metformin. She also sees a nutritionist and a counselor. She is told about the possibility of use of this medication on long-term basis.

She will be prone to have which of the following deficiencies with long-term use of metformin.?

a. Vitamin B1

b. Vitamin B2

c. Vitamin B6

d. Vitamin B12

e. None of the above vitamin deficiency is associated with long-term use of metformin

The correct answer is "d."

Pediatric Obesity—Assessment, Treatment, and Prevention ... academic.oup.com/jcem/article/102/3/709/2965084.

Question 11.15

A 16-year-old girl is started on prescription strength Orlistat to help lose weight. She is also diagnosed with hypothyroidism and takes levothyroxine. She lost 12 pounds in the last 4 months. Her family is very supportive. She has made dietary changes and goes to gym regularly. She presents in the emergency department on one evening with severe right upper quadrant pain. Please select to correct statement.

a. Liver functions need to be monitored

b. Biliary stones can form with the use of orlistat

c. Levothyroxine level may drop with use of orlistat

d. Renal function impairment may be present

e. All the above statements are correct

The correct answer is "e."

All the statements from “a” to “d” are correct.

Pediatric Obesity—Assessment, Treatment, and Prevention ... academic.oup.com/jcem/article/102/3/709/2965084.

Question 11.16

Parents are called for a 12-year-old student about the poor performance in school. The child is hyperactive in class. He does not pay attention to the lessons. He is noted to have disruptive behavior at times. An appointment with the pediatrician is made. Mother reports that kid has a restless sleep most of the days and does frequent bed wetting. His BMI is at 98th percentile for his age. Please select the correct statement regarding the clinical condition of the child.

a. Sleep apnea can be a potential reason for his current symptoms

b. In obese children, tonsils are <u>less</u> commonly the reason for sleep apnea

c. Effective treatment for sleep apnea is not available for pediatric patients

d. There is no difference in Symptoms of adult and Pediatric sleep apnea

e. None of the above statements are correct

The correct answer is "a."

Symptoms of childhood sleep apnea can differ from adults in several respects. Disturbed sleep, snoring, nightmares, and bed wetting can be observed in pediatric patients. Affected kids may be hyperactive as compared to adults with sleep apnea who commonly have sleepiness during the day. Enlarged tonsils can cause obstructive breathing in kids. In overweight children tonsillectomy alone may not alleviate the problem of obstructive sleep apnea.

Huang, Yu-Shu, and Christian Guilleminault. "Pediatric Obstructive Sleep Apnea: Where Do We Stand?" Sleep-Related Breathing Disorders Advances in Oto-Rhino-Laryngology, 2017, pp. 136–144., doi:10.1159/000470885.

Question 11.17

Pediatric NAFLD (Nonalcoholic fatty liver disease) histologically differs from adult NAFLD. Please select the correct statement

a. Pediatric NAFLD shows greater steatosis
b. Pediatric NAFLD has minimal or no hepatocellular ballooning
c. In Pediatric NAFLD there is portal accentuation over zone 3 accentuation
d. All the above statements are correct

Correct answer is "d."

Question 11.18

A 19-years-old girl is found to have insulin resistance. Her BMI is 43. Her insulin level is in range of 35 to 40. She is started on metformin 500 mg orally twice daily. After two day she calls the office complaining of abdominal pain and diarrhea. Please select to correct statement about her condition.

a. Switching to slow-release preparation of metformin may not be helpful
b. Clostridium Difficile infections are common after metformin use
c. Metformin causes bowel ischemia leading to diarrhea and pain
d. Genetic variation may exist regarding side effects and tolerance for metformin

Correct answer is "d."

Slow-release preparation may be better tolerated in some patients. Clostridium Difficile infections have closer association with use of antibiotics. Metformin does not cause bowel ischemia. Genetic variations in metformin intolerance exist and it is an area of interest in research.

McCreight, Laura J et al. "Metformin and the gastrointestinal tract." *Diabetologia* vol. 59,3 (2016): 426-35. doi:10.1007/s00125-015-3844-9

Eating Disorders

Question 12.1

A 25-year-old woman has gained significant weight in last one year. She is seen in the bariatric office. She describes eating an excessive amount of food frequently in a brief time. She frequently feels lack of control and unable to stop once she starts eating. She describes food fantasies before eating episodes. What is the most likely type of disorder expected in her case?

a. Binge eating disorder

b. Compulsive overeating

c. Night eating syndrome

d. Bulimia Nervosa

The correct answer is "b."

Food fantasies and ideation differentiate compulsive overeating from binge eating disorder. Both have shared features of consuming a significant amount of foods very often. The patient is unable to stop and does not fear the consequences of such actions. Binge eating involves feeling of guilt or shame and it is not usually associated with some compensatory acts like purging, excessive exercise or fasting. Bing eating disorder can be mild with 1 to 3 episodes of eating per week. An extreme form can have 14 or more episodes in a week.

https://www.medicinenet.com/compulsive_overeating_vs_binge_eating_disorder/article.htm

Question 12.2

A patient with binge eating disorder is managed in a clinic. The provider opts for the Maudsley method. Which of the following statements is true about this technique of treating Binge eating disorder?

a. Systematic desensitization
b. A compulsory detainment in the hospital is done if the risk of mortality is high.
c. It is a kind of cognitive behavioral therapy
d. It is a type of technique involving family therapy
e. None of the above statements is correct

The correct answer is "d."

Question 12.3

Which of the following statements is correct about bulimia nervosa?

a. It is more common in men
b. It does not involve compensatory behavior to prevent weight gain
c. The altered sensation of smell
d. Deterioration of dental enamel
e. None of the above statements is correct

The correct answer is "d."

Bulimia nervosa is characterized by eating of large amount of food in a discrete period of time, sense of loss of control and inappropriate recurrent compensatory acts to avoid weight gain. These episodes occur at least once per week for 3 months. Repeated acts of vomiting may lead to acid damage to the enamel of teeth. In any suspected case of bulimia, the physician should pay attention to the teeth examination and make proper documentation.

Diagnostic and Statistical Manual of Mental Disorders, Fifth Edition

Question 12.4

Bulimia nervosa is the type of eating disorder which is characterized by binge eating and use of some form of compensatory behavior. Which of the following statements is correct about bulimia nervosa related compensatory behaviors?

a. Using laxatives

b. Exercise

c. Self-induced vomiting

d. All the above statements are correct

e. None of the above statements is correct

The correct answer is "d."

a, b, and c are correct statements as self-induced vomiting, use of laxatives and excessive exercise define the compensatory behaviors to counter the effect of binge eating. It is seen in 1 % of adults and most commonly seen in women. Fluoxetine is an FDA-approved option for treatment of this disorder.

Question 12.5

Which of the following statements is true for patients with Binge eating disorder (BED)?

a. Spontaneous remission is not seen for binge eaters

b. Surgery remains the best tool to manage BED

c. MB-EAT (Mindfulness-based eating disorder training) is part of cognitive behavioral therapy

d. All the above statements are correct

e. None of the above statements is correct

The correct answer is "c."

The BED is considered as an unstable disorder. Spontaneous remission is sometimes seen in BED. Lisdexamfetamine (schedule II) medicine have been approved for the treatment of binge eating disorder.

Fairburn, C. G. (2000). The Natural Course of Bulimia Nervosa and Binge Eating Disorder in Young Women. Archives of

General Psychiatry, 57(7), 659-665.
doi:10.1001/archpsyc.57.7.659

Obesity-Related Issues in Obstetrics and Gynecology

Tawsufe Majid MD and Saima Ashraf MD

Question 13.1

Obesity in women is a common problem contributing to reproductive disadvantages. Select the correct statement.

a. Increased subfertility due to increased insulin resistance
b. Increased risk of first trimester and recurrent miscarriage
c. Increased risk of preterm delivery
d. Increased risk of pregnancies affected by neural tube defects
e. All the above statements are correct

The correct answer is "e."

Obesity is associated with multiple adverse pregnancy outcomes. These include subfertility, recurrent pregnancy loss, preterm delivery and congenital anomalies including neural tube defects.

Editorial Board. (2015). Endocrinology, 156(5). doi: 10.1210/endo.2015.156.issue-5.edboard

Question 13.2

The recommendation for total weight gain during pregnancy for an average weight woman with a BMI of 18.5 to 24.9 is

a. 25 - 35 pounds
b. 35 - 40 pounds
c. 15 - 25 pounds
d. 28 - 40 pounds

The correct answer is “a.”

Recommendations exist for total and rate of weight gain during pregnancy by pre-pregnancy BMI. The recommendation for normal-weight women with a BMI of 18.5 -24.9 is 25-30 pounds. The recommendation for overweight women with a BMI of 25.0 -29.9 is 15 -25 pounds. The recommendation for obese women with a BMI > 30.0 is 1-20 pounds. These recommendations are modified from the Institute of Medicine and National Research Council, 2009.

T Women's Health Care Physicians. (n.d.). Retrieved January 03, 2018, from https://www.acog.org/Clinical-Guidance-and-Publications/Committee-Opinions/Committee-on-Health-Care-for-Underserved-Women/Challenges-for-Overweight-and-Obese-Women

Question 13.3

Maternal obesity is associated with an increased risk for stillbirth when compared with normal weight women. The risk for stillbirth is expected to be higher. Please select the correct statement.

a. 1.0 - 2.0-fold higher compared with normal weight women

b. 2.1 - 4.3-fold higher compared with normal weight women

c. 4.5 - 5.0-fold higher compared with normal weight women

d. 5.0 - 6.5-fold higher compared with normal weight women

The correct answer is "b."

Maternal obesity can affect the fetus. The risks include increased congenital anomalies, growth abnormalities, miscarriage, and stillbirth. The risk for stillbirth is 2.1 – 4.3-fold higher in obese women compared with normal weight women.

PRACTICE BULLETIN - The American Congress of Obstetricians ... (n.d.). Retrieved January 3, 2018

Question 13.4

Which one of the is following is less likely in a morbidly obese pregnant woman?

a. Gestational diabetes
b. Preeclampsia
c. Cesarean section delivery
d. Precipitous delivery

The correct answer is "d."

Gestational diabetes, Preeclampsia, and cesarean section delivery are all increased risks that occur in obese pregnant patients. Rather than precipitous deliveries obese patients are more likely to be admitted earlier in labor, need labor induction, require more oxytocin, and have a longer labor.

Women's Health Care Physicians. (n.d.). Retrieved January 03, 2018, from https://www.acog.org/Resources-And-Publications/Practice-Bulletins-List

Question 13.5

What percentage of women undergoing bariatric surgery are of reproductive age in the United States?

a. 20%

b. 30%

c. 40%

d. 50%

The correct answer is "c."

In the United States, women in reproductive age group represent 40% of patients undergoing bariatric surgery. According to some estimates, 50,000 women of reproductive age undergo bariatric surgery in USA annually.

Editorial Board. (2015). Endocrinology, 156(5). doi: 10.1210/endo.2015.156.issue-5.edboard

Question 13.6

Which one of the following is the least common vitamin deficiencies in obstetric patients who has history of Roux-en-Y gastricbypass?

a. Vitamin C
b. Iron
c. Folate
d. Vitamin D
e. Vitamin B12

The correct answer is "a."

Common nutritional deficiencies after Roux-en-Y gastric bypass surgery include protein, iron, vitamin B12, folate, vitamin D, and calcium.
It is important to recognize specific dietary and micronutrient needs of pregnant women who have undergone Roux-en-Y gastric bypass surgery. Vitamin A needs to be in the form of beta-carotene. 5000 IU is the recommended dose. Vitamin A has teratogenic effects. B12 should be given in a dose of 1mg intramuscular every third month. Thiamine recommendations include 50mg daily. Dose may need to be increased in patient with poor intake with excessive nausea or vomiting. Such patients carry risk of developing Wernicke's encephalopathy. Folic acid recommendation is 400 mcg in first 12 weeks and 5mg in later weeks.
Elevated risk of deficiencies demand monitoring labs to be done in each trimester.

ACOG Practice Bulletin No. 105: Bariatric Surgery and...: Obstetrics & Gynecology. (n.d.). Retrieved January 06, 2018, from http://journals.lww.com/greenjournal/Citation/2009/06000/ACOG_Practice_Bulletin_No__105__Bariatric_Surgery.48.aspx

Question 13.7

Which one of the following is not an option for weight management during pregnancy?

a. Dietary control
b. Anorectics
c. Exercise
d. Behavior modification

The correct answer is "b."

The primary weight management strategies during pregnancy are dietary control, exercise, and behavior modification. Medications for weight management are not recommended during the time of conception or pregnancy because of safety concerns and adverse effects.

Editorial Board. (2015). Endocrinology, 156(5). doi: 10.1210/endo.2015.156.issue-5.edboard

Question 13.8

Morbidly obese patients pose several management challenges in obstetrics and gynecology practice. Certain interesting trends have been observed about higher BMI. The "Obesity Paradox" refers to

a. Overall, lower mortality and composite morbidity in the obese patient without metabolic complications than that of a healthy weight patient undergoing general surgery.
b. Overall higher mortality and composite morbidity in the obese patient without metabolic complications than that of a healthy weight patient undergoing general surgery.
c. Overall higher mortality and composite morbidity in the obese patient with metabolic complications than that of a healthy weight patient undergoing general surgery

The correct answer is "a"

A prospective, multi-institutional, risk-adjusted cohort study of 118,707 patients who underwent non-bariatric general surgery examined mortality risks and found the highest rates in the underweight and morbidly obese extremes and the lowest rates in the overweight and moderately obese. Obese patients with metabolic syndrome (specifically, hypertension and diabetes) who undergo general, vascular, and orthopedic surgery are at increased risk of perioperative morbidity and mortality compared with normal weight patients.

Committee Opinion No. 619. (2015). Obstetrics & Gynecology, 125(1), 274-278. doi:10.1097/01.aog.0000459870.06491.71

Question 13.9

The American College of Obstetricians and Gynecologist makes the recommendations based on expert opinion and available data. Which of the following statements is correct?

a. The evidence demonstrates that, in general, vaginal hysterectomy is associated with better outcomes and fewer complications than laparoscopic or abdominal hysterectomy

b. Preoperative consultation with an anesthesiologist should be considered for the obese patient in whom the possibility of obstructive sleep apnea is suspected on clinical grounds or who is at risk of CAD, has a difficult airway, or has poorly controlled hypertension.

c. Preoperative imaging (e.g., magnetic resonance imaging etc.) may help to determine the best route of surgery in obese patients.

d. All the above statements are correct

The correct answer is "d."

All the above are ACOG recommendations. Preoperative imaging may be beneficial because the office abdominal and bimanual examination may be difficult in obese patients.

Committee Opinion No. 619. (2015). Obstetrics & Gynecology, 125(1), 274-278. doi:10.1097/01.aog.0000459870.06491.71

Question 13.10

Obese patients undergoing gynecologic procedures longer than 45 minutes, and not at risk of major bleeding fall into what risk category for venous thromboembolism?

a. Very low-risk patients
b. Low-risk patients
c. Moderate risk patients
d. High-risk patients

The correct answer is "c."

Obese patients undergoing gynecologic procedures longer than 45 minutes and not at risk of major bleeding, fall into the category of moderate risk of venous thromboembolism. Moderate risk surgical patients have been defined as those with a Caprini's score of 3 to 4. Their estimated baseline risk of venous thromboembolic disease (VTD) in the absence of prophylaxis is 3 percent. Moderate risk patients should receive prophylaxis in the form of low molecular weight heparin, low dose unfractionated heparin, or mechanical prophylaxis with intermittent pneumatic compression

Committee Opinion No. 619. (2015). Obstetrics & Gynecology, 125(1), 274-278. doi:10.1097/01.aog.0000459870.06491.71

Question 13.11

Respiratory morbidity is more common in the obese patient. Post-operative hypoxemia can be addressed by the following measures EXCEPT

a. Use of aggressive incentive spirometry
b. Use of continuous positive airway pressure
c. Conservative use of postoperative opioids
d. Avoidance of nonsteroidal anti-inflammatory drugs administered preoperatively or intraoperatively

The correct answer is "d."

Nonsteroidal anti-inflammatory drugs administered preoperatively or intraoperatively appear to be more effective than acetaminophen in reducing nausea and vomiting and total post-operative opioid use.

The American College of Obstetricians and Gynecologist COMMITTEE OPINION Number 619, January 2015, Gynecologic Surgery in the Obese Woman.

Question 13.12

Long-term follow up of the offspring of obese women can show some disorders in later life. Which of the following statements is correct?

a. Increased risk of childhood obesity
b. Decreased risk of autism spectrum disorders
c. Decreased risk of childhood asthma

The correct answer is "a."

There are long-term risks to the offspring of obese women. These include increased risk of metabolic syndrome, childhood obesity, autism spectrum disorders, and childhood asthma. On the other hand, maternal malnutrition during early pregnancy can lead to higher risk of developing obesity in the child in later life.

Editorial Board. (2015). Endocrinology, 156(5). doi:10.1210/endo.2015.156.issue-5.edboard

Question 13.13

Pregnancy outcomes in women after bariatric surgery compared with obese and morbidly obese controls indicate some difference. Please select the correct statement.

a. Bariatric surgery is associated with a reduction in the rate of gestational diabetes in a subsequent pregnancy
b. There is a significant difference in the rate of hypertensive disorders of pregnancy after bariatric surgery
c. Neonates were significantly less likely to be small for gestational age in the bariatric surgery group

The correct answer is "a."

There was a significant decrease in the rate of gestational diabetes in bariatric surgery patients (0.0%) as compared with both control groups (morbidly obese 16.4%, obese 9.3%). There was no significant difference in the rate of hypertensive disorders of pregnancy with bariatric surgery. Additionally, neonates were significantly more likely to be small for gestational age (SGA) in the bariatric surgery group.

Lesko, J., & Peaceman, A. (2012). Pregnancy Outcomes in Women After Bariatric Surgery Compared With Obese and Morbidly Obese Controls. Obstetrics & Gynecology, 119(3), 547-554. doi:10.1097/aog.0b013e318239060e

Question 13.14

The association of body mass index, operative time and perioperative morbidity after hysterectomy varies among abdominal, laparoscopic, and vaginal approaches. Which of the following associations have been observed?

a. Women undergoing abdominal hysterectomy who had BMIs 40 or higher when compared to women with a normal BMI had five times the odds of wound dehiscence

b. The magnitude of the association between wound infection and BMI was smaller after vaginal hysterectomy

c. Operative time increased with BMI regardless of surgical approach

d. All the above are correct

The correct answer is "d."

Obesity is associated with increased wound complications and infections in women undergoing an abdominal hysterectomy and with more extended operative times regardless of the surgical approach. Vaginal or laparoscopic hysterectomy should be performed whenever feasible.

Shah, D. K., Vitonis, A. F., & Missmer, S. A. (2015). Association of Body Mass Index and Morbidity After Abdominal, Vaginal, and Laparoscopic Hysterectomy. Obstetrics & Gynecology, 125(3), 589-598. doi:10.1097/aog.0000000000000698

Question 13.15

Late complications of previous bariatric surgery have occurred during pregnancy. These include the following.

a. Maternal intestinal obstruction
b. Gastrointestinal hemorrhage
c. Cholelithiasis
d. All above are correct

The correct answer is "d."

Several case reports and small studies have identified significant late complications of previous bariatric surgery that have occurred during pregnancy. These include maternal intestinal obstruction and gastrointestinal hemorrhage. Exploratory surgery during pregnancy may be required to treat these complications from bariatric surgery.

The American College of Obstetrics and Gynecologist Practice Bulletin, Number 105, June 2009 (Reaffirmed 2017), Bariatric Surgery and Pregnancy

Question 13.16

A 27-year-old female who is eighteen weeks gravida presents to the ER with excessive vomiting for the last one week. The patient had adjustable gastric band surgery in the past for obesity. The previous fill for the band was done six months ago. She does not have any other significant comorbidities. Initial evaluation in the emergency room shows signs of dehydration. Her blood pressure is 110/ 70 with a heart rate of 86. Imaging study shows that band is in position with calculation of phi angle close to 40°. She is initially managed with IV fluids and antiemetics. What can be the additional appropriate strategy regarding her management?

a. Adjustable gastric band should be removed immediately as it has likely slipped

b. Deflation of the band should be done through the access port

c. A barium small bowel follow-through study should be carried out

d. Topiramate may be started to prevent weight gain after deflation of band.

The correct answer is "b."

Deflation of the band should be done in this case. Topiramate has no role in acute condition as stated in the question. Topiramate is highly teratogenic. Its use is contraindicated in this setting. Surgery may be considered as a last resort in cases of band slippage with severe gastric outlet obstruction which is not relieved with deflation. Surgery is also a consideration if erosion of band in the stomach is discovered. Transverse position on X-ray study points to a possible slipped band. A phi angle determination is useful. It is calculated by drawing a vertical line to parallel to the vertebral column and second line through the long axis of the band. The angle is measured where both lines cross. Normally it is in the range of 4° to 58°. It is important to compare the angle with previous imaging studies in the same patient.

Knipe, Henry. "Slipped Gastric Band | Radiology Case." Radiopaedia.org, radiopaedia.org/cases/slipped-gastric-band.

Question 13.17

A morbidly obese 30-year-old female is referred to her OB/GYN physician for counseling of appropriate birth control options. She has been on combination oral contraceptive pill regimen. She is also following with a bariatric practice. She is using Topiramate phentermine combination for the last couple of months for weight loss. Which of the following statements is correct?

a. The patient may experience breakthrough bleeding
b. Ethinyl estradiol levels may become lower by 30% with concurrent topiramate use
c. Ethinyl estradiol levels may become higher by 30% with concurrent topiramate use
d. Ethinyl estradiol levels are not changed with concurrent topiramate use
e. Norethindrone levels are increased by 50% with concurrent topiramate use

f. a and b are correct

The correct answer is "f."

It has been observed that levels of estrogen component of oral contraceptive pills may become lower with concurrent use of topiramate. This can result in breakthrough bleedings.

Rosenfeld, W. E., Doose, D. R., Walker, S. A., & Nayak, R. K. (1997). Effect of Topiramate on the Pharmacokinetics of an Oral Contraceptive Containing Norethindrone and Ethinyl Estradiol in Patients with Epilepsy. Epilepsia, 38(3), 317-323. doi:10.1111/j.1528-1157.1997.tb01123.x

Question 13.18

24-year-old female patient who is gravida 0 presents with complaints of oligomenorrhea, excessive facial hair and weight gain. Physical exam shows BMI 41, hirsutism, acanthosis nigricans, abdominal striae with large pannus, and Tanner's stage IV development. Workup shows negative urine pregnancy test, elevated HbA1C, elevated fasting blood sugar, deranged lipid profile, elevated fasting serum insulin, elevated free testosterone, normal DHEAS, normal 17 hydroxyprogesterone acetate, normal TSH and normal prolactin. 24-hour urinary free cortisol excretion test is normal. Please select which of the following differential diagnoses is suspected?

a. Adrenal hyperplasia

b. PCOS (polycystic ovarian syndrome)

c. Cushing's syndrome

d. Hypothyroidism

e. Hyperprolactinemia

The correct answer is "b."

Question 13.19

What would be the next management steps in the case discussed above?

a. Pelvic ultrasound

b. Progesterone challenge followed by combined birth control pills

c. Metformin

d. Counseling about weight loss and healthy lifestyle

e. All the above statements are correct

The correct answer is "e."

Question 13.20

The above patient followed up in the office after three months. She now has regular menstrual cycles. She has not been able to lose significant weight. The patient is counseled about the importance of losing weight and its potential benefits. She is told that there is a possibility of a positive impact on her reproductive and metabolic abnormalities if she can lose 10 % or more of her excess weight. Select the correct statement regarding her further management

a. Referral to a bariatric surgery practice
b. Consideration for the use of weight loss medications
c. Counseling about birth control options if she chooses to use a phentermine-topiramate combination
d. Continue nutritional counseling and follow up
e. All the above statements

The correct answer is "e."

Question 13.21

A 35-year-old female patient who is gravida 0 with Class III obesity and primary infertility is followed in the OBGYN office. Patient has been evaluated for infertility, and she is diagnosed with ovulatory factor infertility and PCOS. Patient has failed multiple trials of ovulation induction.
The patient is currently on Levo-thyroxine and Metformin. She decided to have bariatric surgery procedure before attempting to get pregnant. How long should a patient wait after bariatric surgery before attempting pregnancy?

a. 3 – 6 months
b. 6 – 9 months
c. 9 – 12 months

d. More than one year

The correct answer is "d."

Question 13.22

What are the recommendations for screening for diabetes in pregnancy in patients who have undergone bariatric surgery?

a. 50 g 1-hour glucose tolerance test (GTT) at 26 to 28 weeks
b. 100 g 3-hour GTT at 26 to 28 weeks
c. 75 g 2-hour GTT at 26 to 28 weeks
d. Fasting and 1-hour postprandial blood sugars for one week at 24 to 26 weeks

The correct answer is "d."

Question 13.23

Obese pregnant women are at increased risk for several complications. Select the correct statement.

a. Cesarean delivery
b. Endometritis
c. Wound dehiscence

d. Venous thrombosis

e. All the above are correct

The correct answer is "e."

All the complications stated above occur more frequently in obese pregnant patients.

Question 13.24

Neonates of obese mothers are at increased risk of all EXCEPT

a. Neonatal injury during delivery

b. Neural tube defects

c. Limb reduction anomalies

d. Gastroschisis

e. Cardiovascular anomalies

The correct answer is "d."

Question 13.25

A 24-year-old female G4P2 at 28 weeks gestation, is sent to OB triage from her PCP office with chief complaints of persistent vomiting and abdominal pain. Past medical history is significant for asthma, PCOS, anemia, rheumatoid arthritis, and obesity. Past surgical history includes two cesarean sections, gastric bypass surgery (done two years ago), and

history of first trimester vaginal bleeding which resolved spontaneously.
On examination maternal tachycardia is noted. She is afebrile and lungs are clear on auscultation.
Abdomen: Gravid, generalized tenderness with guarding

Pelvic exam: cervical os closed with no bleeding or leakage of fluids.
Initial workup shows white blood count of 18000, CMP: Na 138 mEq/L, K 4.1 mEq/L, BUN 26, Creatinine 0.6 mg/dl, AST 13, ALT 14, Amylase 24, and Lipase 12. Urine analysis shows 2+ blood and 3+ketones. OB ultrasound shows normal fetal parameters and some fluid in the pelvis. Fetal heart tracings are normal. There is no evidence of contractions on CTG (cardiotocograph). In her case differential diagnosis includes all the following EXCEPT

a. Preterm labor
b. Acute Cholecystitis
c. Acute Pancreatitis
d. Chorioamnionitis
e. Placental abruption
f. Cesarean scar dehiscence
g. Perforated marginal ulcer at gastrojejunostomy
h. UTI
i. Appendicitis

The correct answer is “a.”

Any surgical complications as stated above can occur in pregnant women. It poses diagnostic and management challenges. A high index of suspicion is needed in post-gastric bypass patients. Complications like internal hernias or perforated ulcers can mimic many other acute intraabdominal pathologies. There is a high risk of complications in these scenarios. Rarely, pancreatitis can exist with normal related enzyme levels.

Question 13.26

Bariatric surgery can alter the course of pregnancy and outcome. Please select the correct statement.

a. There is a lower incidence of severe obesity in children in later life, born to mothers having successful bariatric surgery
b. There is no change in the incidence of gestational diabetes in mothers who had bariatric surgery versus those who did not.
c. Microcephaly is noted more frequently in babies born to mothers who had bariatric surgery
d. Birth length of babies born to mothers who had bariatric surgery is less as compared to babies born to mother who did not have bariatric surgery.
e. All the above statements are correct

The correct answer is "a."

Low birth weights have been observed in babies born to mothers who had bariatric procedures in the past. There has not been a significant difference in birth length and head

circumference. There are strong recommendations about monitoring of various nutrients during gestations. Iron, B12, folic acid, Hemoglobin, and serum albumin needs special attention. Hypoproteinemia can be a concern in malabsorptive procedures like a duodenal switch and gastric bypass.
Pregnancy outcomes and nutritional indices after three types of bariatric surgery 2014 Nov Dec Soard.

Question 13.27

A 23-year-old female is seeing her family physician for annual physical. She is thinking to start oral contraceptives for birth control. She has concerns about weight gain with the use of this type of contraception. Please select the correct statement.

a. Current oral contraceptives have a great potential to cause weight gain due to estrogen content
b. Fat storage is more likely than fluid retention to cause weight gain with use of oral contraceptives
c. Older contraceptives had high estrogen content, and these were more likely to cause weight gain.
d. Progesterone component of oral contraceptives is a likely factor in causing weight gain

The correct answer is "c."

Older oral contraceptives which were available several decades ago, had very high estrogen content. These led to weight gain by increasing hunger and fluid retention. Current generation of oral contraceptives have low estrogens. These are not thought to cause significant weight gain. Any patient using these medications should be aware of these facts. Dietary counseling may help in the patients prone to gain weight.

Orthopedics and Obesity

Question 14.1

When considering the timeline of performing bariatric surgery in respect to a total shoulder replacement in morbidly obese patients, what is the appropriate sequence of performing bariatric surgery?

a. Bariatric surgery should be performed before a total shoulder replacement
b. Bariatric surgery should be performed after a total shoulder replacement
c. The timing of bariatric surgery has no relevance
d. Bariatric surgery and total shoulder replacement surgery should be performed concurrently

The correct answer is "a."
A review of the Medicare database on 300 patients who underwent bariatric surgery prior or after a total shoulder replacement surgery showed that there were higher rates of prosthesis instability (7.9%) and loosening (8.6%) in patients who had bariatric surgery after a total shoulder replacement. The rate of hardware prosthesis/loosening were 4.8(4.2%) in patients who had a bariatric surgery before a total shoulder replacement surgery and 5.1(4.9%) in patients who just a total shoulder replacement. The findings of this study support that it should be considered to perform bariatric surgery prior to a total shoulder replacement in the morbidly obese patient as opposed to after.

Cancienne JM, Camp CL, Brockmeier SF, Gulotta LV, Dines DM, Werner BC. Bariatric Surgery Following Total Shoulder Arthroplasty Increases the Risk for Mechanical Complications Including Instability and Prosthetic Loosening. HSS Journal®. 2018 Jul 1;14(2):108-13.

Question 14.2

Which risk factor is associated with an elevated risk for morbidity and readmission following knee, hip, and shoulder arthroscopy?

a. Female Gender
b. Participation in contact sports
c. Class III obesity with diabetes mellitus
d. Family history of hypertension and coronary artery disease

The correct answer is "c."
A review of 140,000 patients who underwent elective knee, hip, or shoulder arthroscopy was conducted assessing rates of morbidity, mortality, readmission, reoperation, and venous thromboembolism using univariate analyses and binary logistic regression between patients with or without diabetes mellitus and body mass index. Class III obesity with diabetes was a risk factor for morbidity (odds ratio [OR] = 1.522; 95% confidence interval [CI], 1.101-2.103) and readmission (OR = 2.342; 95% CI, 1.998-2.745) following all procedures.

Nicolay RW, Selley RS, Terry MA, Tjong VK. Body Mass Index as a Risk Factor for 30-Day Postoperative Complications in Knee, Hip, and Shoulder Arthroscopy. Arthroscopy: The Journal of Arthroscopic & Related Surgery. 2019 Feb 4.

Question 14.3

According to recent literature, which pre-operative parameter is more predictive of clinical, and patient reported knee and hip function outcomes post-total joint arthroplasty?

a. Body Mass Index
b. Percent Body Fat
c. Hemoglobin A1C
d. Degree of loss of knee flexion

The correct answer is "b."
A prospective study of 215 patients who underwent either a total knee or hip arthroplasty was conducted following the patients up to 2 years with the University of California, Los Angeles (UCLA). The activity scale; the Knee Injury and Osteoarthritis Outcome Score (KOOS) for total knee arthroplasty; and the Hip Disability and Osteoarthritis Outcome Score (HOOS) for total hip arthroplasty were monitored. The results of this study showed that higher percent of body fat predicted the occurrence of surgical complications.

Ledford CK, Millikan PD, Nickel BT, Green CL, Attarian DE, Wellman SS, Bolognesi MP, Queen RM. Percent body fat is more predictive of function after total joint arthroplasty than body mass index. JBJS. 2016 May 18;98(10):849-57.

Question 14.4

What outcomes have not been shown to change post-operatively up to 5 years from a total ankle reconstruction surgery?

a. Pain
b. Ankle Function
c. Body Mass Index
d. Quality of Life

The correct answer is "c."
According to a retrospective review of 145 overweight and obese patients, pain and disability significantly reduce after ankle replacement or fusion surgery. However, mean body mass index remains unchanged from an ankle reconstruction surgery in the overweight and obese patients.

Penner MJ, Pakzad H, Younger A, Wing KJ. Mean BMI of overweight and obese patients does not decrease after successful ankle reconstruction. JBJS. 2012 May 2;94(9):e57.

Question 14.5

There are many challenges faced by super-obese patients with a BMI > 50.0 kg/m2 after total hip arthroplasty. Which of the following is not true?

a. Increased risk of revision
b. Lower implant survival
c. Difficulty finding an orthopedic surgeon to operate
d. Large implant required

The correct answer is "d."

A case-control study comparing super-obese patients and matched non-obese patients showed that super-obese patients are 4.5 times more likely to undergo a revision, with an 89.6% of implant survival and report inferior patient reported outcomes. Super-obese patients were also evaluated by a larger number of orthopedic surgeons prior to surgery.

Issa K, Harwin SF, Malkani AL, Bonutti PM, Scillia A, Mont MA. Bariatric orthopedics: total hip arthroplasty in super-obese patients (those with a BMI of≥ 50 kg/m2). JBJS. 2016 Feb 3;98(3):180-5.

Question 14.6

Which statement concerning the prevalence of slipped capital femoral epiphysis (SCFE) in obese children is true?

a. SCFE is highly prevalent in obese children at an earlier age compared to non-obese children.
b. Obese children have a higher prevalence of unilateral SCFE compared to non-obese children.
c. The reported evidence of SCFE in obese children is decreasing.
d. SCFE does not require surgical intervention.

The correct answer is "a."
Recent literature presents that SCFE is beginning to be more common especially in obese children requiring surgical pinning. The clinical presentation in the obese children is usually bilateral disease.

Azzopardi T, Sharma S, Bennet GC. Slipped capital femoral epiphysis in children aged less than 10 years. Journal of Pediatric Orthopedics B. 2010 Jan 1;19(1):13-8.

Question 14.7

Which co-morbidity should be screened and treated prior to an orthopedic surgical procedure?

a. Obstructive Sleep Apnea
b. Stroke
c. Peripheral arterial disease
d. Varicose veins

The correct answer is "a."
Obstructive sleep apnea (OSA) is a common condition screened before bariatric surgery. OSA is a factor for post-operative morbidity and mortality i.e., pulmonary embolism, wound complications, etc. An 8-item questionnaire called the STOP BANG can help assess for the risk of OSA. It treatment may include supplemental oxygen or a continuous positive airway pressure machine after surgery.

Mihalko WM, Bergin PF, Kelly FB, Canale ST. Obesity, orthopaedics, and outcomes. JAAOS-Journal of the American Academy of Orthopaedic Surgeons. 2014 Nov 1;22(11):683-90.

Question 14.8

Obesity has been known to misalign the knee. What position promotes medial compartment knee osteoarthrosis?

a. Genu Valgus
b. Genu Varus
c. Genu Recurvatum
d. Patella Baja

The correct answer is "b."

A cross-sectional study on 300 patients with knee osteoarthritis showed that BMI clinically and statistically correlated with osteoarthritis severity in patients with genu varus but not in genu valgus.
Sharma L, Lou C, Cahue S, Dunlop DD. The mechanism of the effect of obesity in knee osteoarthritis: the mediating role of malalignment. Arthritis & Rheumatism: Official Journal of the American College of Rheumatology. 2000 Mar;43(3):568-75.

Question 14.9

What strategies can a morbidly obese patient take prior to undergoing elective orthopedic surgery?

a. Undergo a psychiatric consultation
b. Hypnotization therapy to reduce hunger and disordered eating habits
c. Participate in a weight-loss program
d. Outcomes from an elective orthopedic surgery is the same for morbid obese and non-obese patients

The correct answer is "c."
The American Academy of Orthopedic Surgeons (AAOS) released a position statement on obesity, bone, and joint health. The AAOS recommends the following for morbidly obese patients before an elective orthopedic surgery:

- Discuss with their physician about how to lose weight and the impact of weight on the surgery outcomes.
- Delay the surgery.
- Develop a plan to manage comorbidities.
- Perform a nutritional assessment.
- Discuss the rehabilitation protocol after surgery.
- Have the patient sign a commitment form to lose weight, eat healthier and exercise after surgery.
- Participate in a weight-loss program.

The Impact of Obesity on Bone and Joint Health Women M, Ranges BM. The Impact of Obesity on Bone and Joint Health.

Question 14.10

What is not an independent risk for plantar fasciitis?

a. Reduced ankle dorsiflexion
b. Obesity
c. Work-related weight-bearing
d. Limb length

The correct answer is "d."
A case-control study was performed to examine the risk factors for plantar fasciitis. Patients who had an ankle dorsiflexion angle less than 0 degrees, BMI > 30 kg/m2 and occupations requiring working on their feet had an odds ratio of 23.3, 5.6, and 3.6, respectively compared to the group that did not have those factors i.e., ankle dorsiflexion angle >10 degrees, BMI < 25 kg/m2, etc.

Riddle DL, Pulisic M, Pidcoe P, Johnson RE. Risk factors for plantar fasciitis: a matched case-control study. JBJS. 2003 May 1;85(5):872-7.

Question 14.11

A 42-year-old female who is one year post sleeve gastrectomy presents with progressive weakness of left lower extremity. She lost about 110 lbs. Physical examination reveals left foot drop. Lab work show normal vitamin levels.

Please select the correct statement.

a. Tibial nerve pathology is likely present
b. Femoral nerve involvement is likely

c. Common peroneal nerve damage could be a likely reason
d. Ultrasound is best test to identify the problem

Correct answer is "c."

Extensive weight loss may lead to loss of protective fat making common peroneal nerve prone to compression. It is postulated that changes in fascial tissues could also be contributory. Management requires a close follow up. Vitamin levels need to be checked. Vitamins B12, D, E, folic acid, and copper deficiencies have been associated with neuropathies. These deficiencies however lead more likely to polyneuropathy. MRI scan can be used to detect loss of pad of fat at fibular neck area. About one fourth of such cases have been treated medically and rest have required surgical decompression of nerve.

Lale A, Kirkil C, Ozturk S, Yur M, Can OF, Artaş G, Aygen E. The results of surgical decompression in the treatment of foot drop due to peroneal nerve entrapment after bariatric surgery. Surg Obes Relat Dis. 2020 Nov;16(11):1684-1691. doi: 10.1016/j.soard.2020.06.054. Epub 2020 Jul 15. PMID: 32800521.

Book Page

https://www.facebook.com/MedicalFronts

For List of Errata Visit

https://obesityreviewmultiplechoicequestions.blogspot.com/2019/01/obesity-qeustions.html

Subscribe to Newsletter

https://medicalfronts.com/index.php/subscribe-to-newsletter/

Obesity Insights and Learning: Self-Assessment Exam

(Another resource to practice obesity questions)

https://medicalfronts.com/index.php/obesity-insights-and-learning/

Made in the USA
Coppell, TX
05 November 2023